FINANCING HEALTH CARE IN THE 1990s

John Appleby

Open University Press
Buckingham · Philadelphia

Open University Press
Celtic Court
22 Ballmoor
Buckingham
MK18 1XW

and
1900 Frost Road, Suite 101
Bristol, PA 19007, USA

First Published 1992
Reprinted 1993

A catalogue record of this book is available from the British Library

Library of Congress Cataloging-in-Publication Data

Appleby, John, 1958–
Financing healthcare in the 1990's/John Appleby.
p. cm. – (Open University Press state of health series)
Includes bibliographical references and index.
ISBN 0–335–09776–6 (pb.) ISBN 0–335–09777–4 (hb.)
1. Medical economics – Great Britain. 2. National Health Service (Great Britain) I. Title. II. Title: Financing health care in the 1990's III. Series: State of health series.
[DNLM: 1. Delivery of Health Care – economics – Great Britain. 2. Financing, Government – Great Britain. 3. Health Care Costs – trends – Great Britain. 4. State Medicine – economics – Great Britain W 84 FA1 A6f]
RA410.55.G7A66 1992
338.4'33621'0941 – dc20
DNLM/DLC
for Library of Congress 91–46375
CIP

Typeset by Type Study, Scarborough
Printed in Great Britain by St Edmundsbury Press
Bury St Edmunds, Suffolk

FINANCING HEALTH CARE IN THE 1990s

Department of Social Policy and Social Work
University of Oxford
Barnett House
32 Wellington Square
Oxford OX1 2ER
England

STATE OF HEALTH SERIES

Edited by Chris Ham, Director of Health Services Management Centre, University of Birmingham

Current and forthcoming titles

Financing Health Care in the 1990s
John Appleby

Patients, Policies and Politics
John Butler

Going Private
Michael Calnan, Sarah Cant and Jonathan Gabe

Implementing GP Fundholding: Wild Card or Winning Hand?
Howard Glennerster, Manos Matsaganis and Patricia Owens with Stephanie Hancock

Controlling Health Professionals
Stephen Harrison and Christopher Pollitt

Managing Scarcity
Rudolf Klein, Patricia Day and Sharon Redmayne

Public Law and Health Service Accountability
Diane Longley

Hospitals in Transition
Tim Packwood, Justin Keen and Martin Buxton

The Incompetent Doctor: Behind Closed Doors
Marilynn M. Rosenthal

Planned Markets and Public Competition
Richard B. Saltman and Casten von Otter

Implementing Planned Markets in Health Care
Richard B. Saltman and Caster von Otter (Eds)

Accreditation: Protecting the Professional or the Consumer?
Ellie Scrivens

Whose Standards? Consumer and Professional Standards in Health Care
Charlotte Williamson

CONTENTS

SERIES EDITOR'S INTRODUCTION

Health services in many developed countries have come under critical scrutiny in recent years. In part this is because of increasing expenditure, much of it funded from public sources, and the pressure this has put on governments seeking to control public spending. Also important has been the perception that resources allocated to health services are not always deployed in an optimal fashion. Thus at a time when the scope for increasing expenditure is extremely limited, there is a need to search for ways of using existing budgets more efficiently. A further concern has been the desire to ensure access to health care of various groups on an equitable basis. In some countries this has been linked to a wish to enhance patient choice and to make service providers more responsive to patients as 'consumers'.

Underlying these specific concerns are a number of more fundamental developments which have a significant bearing on the performance of health services. Three are worth highlighting. First, there are demographic changes, including the ageing population and the decline in the proportion of the population of working age. These changes will both increase the demand for health care and at the same time limit the ability of health services to respond to this demand.

Second, advances in medical science will also give rise to new demands within the health services. These advances cover a range of possibilities, including innovations in surgery, drug therapy, screening and diagnosis. The pace of innovation is likely to quicken as the end of the century approaches, with significant implications for the funding and provision of services.

Third, public expectations of health services are rising as those who use services demand higher standards of care. In part, this is stimulated by developments within the health service, including the availability of new technology. More fundamentally, it stems from the emergence of a more educated and informed population, in which people are accustomed to being treated as consumers rather than patients.

Against this background, policymakers in a number of countries are reviewing the future of health services. Those countries which have traditionally relied on a market in health care are making greater use of regulation and planning. Equally, those countries which have traditionally relied on regulation and planning are moving towards a more competitive approach. In no country is there complete satisfaction with existing methods of financing and delivery, and everywhere there is a search for new policy instruments.

The aim of this series is to contribute to debate about the future of health services through an analysis of major issues in health policy. These issues have been chosen because they are both of current interest and of enduring importance. The series is intended to be accessible to students and informed lay readers as well as to specialists working in this field. The aim is to go beyond a textbook approach to health policy analysis and to encourage authors to move debate about their issue forward. In this sense, each book presents a summary of current research and thinking, and an exploration of future policy directions.

Professor Chris Ham
Director of Health Services Management Centre,
University of Birmingham

PREFACE

The UK National Health Service (NHS) has embarked on a potentially massive change in the way it provides health care. How that health care is financed over the coming decade, and how the method of financing dictates (and is in turn dictated to by) the way the UK's health-care system is organized and run will affect us all. Will the Government's stated commitment to a health-care system financed mainly out of general taxation remain? Or, if the current reforms fail to bring measurable benefits of any significance, will the political pressures to take the reforms even further lead to major changes in funding and financing of health care in this country? Will external influences in the economy at large necessitate further reforms of health care? Or perhaps the current reforms will take an unexpected path with some unexpected outcomes?

This book explores some of the directions that health care, in particular the financing of health care, could take over the next ten years. The first chapter introduces the context to the prospects for financing health care in the 1990s, and outlines some of the issues which make health-care financing such an important factor influencing the way health services will be organized and delivered in the future. Subsequent chapters review some of the basic issues in financing such as levels of funding, past trends in funding, systems of financing – from free to managed markets – drawing on international experiences and present some views of the future of health-care financing in the UK as a result of the recently introduced reforms of the NHS.

Although we all have an interest in health and health care, this does not always extend to the intricate details of accounting procedures, resource allocation formulae or the complicated theoretical underpinnings of utility or welfare maximization, etc. Whilst these and other issues are raised in this book, an attempt has been made to do so in an accessible way, and not to obscure the larger issues which are, or should be, of concern to all of us. It is hoped that the book will be of interest to those working in the health service, studying social administration, working in government or public-sector finance and others concerned with the current evolution of the NHS. This last group should especially include the users of health care – which, at one time or other, includes all of us, not only as patients but as taxpayers and, as that oft quoted group in whose interest politicians and others act, the public.

1

NEW DIRECTIONS

SETTING SAIL

In this first year of the reforms in the UK (1991–92), the National Health Service (NHS), like a superliner slipped from its moorings, took time to gather momentum. And for patients and taxpayers, change appeared minimal. In fact, 'stability clauses' introduced into the operation of the reforms in their first year guaranteed that change was kept to an absolute minimum. Previous years' patient flow patterns and services were essentially maintained with changes only allowed at the margin. But the superliner will gather speed. The course it will take is confused, however. There are many pilots offering advice to the captain as to the best way out of the harbour and many others trying to get their hands on the wheel.

Everyone on board seems to have a more or less agreed notion of their destination – those fabled islands of Efficiency and Equality. There is some disagreement over what these islands look like or whether it will be possible to berth at both simultaneously. Some of the crew and many of the passengers are muttering. Some of the crew jump ship to the sleek (but half empty) speed boats bound for the land of Profit. Some of the passengers disembark for the superior cabin service and personalized quoit sticks of the speed boats. There, they get to sit at the captain's table. And the ship's doctors smile as they prescribe pills for seasickness.

For many of the passengers on board the fact that the ship has set sail has gone completely unnoticed. And for most the reason for setting sail in the first place is a mystery. But others support the crew as they confront the captain with demands for guarantees – such as no reduction in the number of deckchairs. The ship's officers are secretly excited, however. This is their chance! For years they have overseen the tugs pulling the ship up and down the river, but now they actually have an opportunity to sail the ship on the open seas. The captain appears confident. Amidst the arguments and near mutinies, he proclaims that whilst a bit low on fuel and still with some excess baggage, the Trade Winds will speed the ship and the rush of the water will clean the hull of its impeding detritus and barnacles.

Analogies, like supertankers, tend to gather considerable speed and a momentum of their own once started, and then take some time to stop. However, the NHS as a ship analogy, setting off into unchartered waters, with only half a wheel (only tenuously connected to the rudder), a crew who speak different languages (and have just been told they must learn a new one), with some of the passengers asked to supplement the underpowered engines by taking to the oars, is not a picture which will go unrecognized by many concerned with and about the NHS.

Evidence for a reformed NHS

In January 1988, the then Prime Minister, Margaret Thatcher pledged to implement a review of the NHS. *Sotto voce* murmurings of such a review were to be heard during the previous year. Many organizations – following a lead by the Institute of Health Services Management (1989) – embarked on their own reviews of the NHS. The year 1988 was also the fortieth anniversary of the NHS. Some felt that it was experiencing a crisis of middle age and was in need of a new direction, a new purpose. Some saw the NHS not as a successful institution but merely as the next lumbering, inefficient bureaucracy requiring the cleansing and efficiency-inducing catharsis of market competition – much like British Telecom, British Gas and Cable & Wireless.

Although many professed surprise at the Prime Minister's apparently spontaneous NHS reform pledge, there is evidence that active and extensive consideration of reform of the NHS started much earlier. In 1981 the then Secretary of State for Health asked civil servants at the Department of Health to organize a working party (set up in July 1981) to investigate alternative ways of financing the NHS. The working party was expressly directed to identify,

(a) alternative sources of finance for the NHS, including different forms of social and private insurance, new and higher charges, and any other forms of payments or contributions by individuals or groups.

(b) alternative ways of promoting more private sector provision of services, including tax concessions (on investment or private insurance), contracting out the state insurance, reimbursement of treatment costs and discontinuing parts of the NHS.

These formed part of the terms of reference for the working group which produced its initial report (Report of the Working Party on Alternative Means of Financing Health Care) in late 1981. Further work was carried out by this group which, as their original terms of reference stated, 'might form the basis of a Green Paper later that year [1982]'. In fact, the seeds of change can probably be traced back in one form or another to the very inception of the NHS. What was perhaps different in the early 1980s was the existence of a Government committed to radical change for the public sector. The NHS's immunity from the reforms going on around it in the rest of the public sector in the 1980s derived partly from its popularity amongst the public as an institution. Reforming the NHS would not be an easy political option. This option was perhaps made easier, however, by the financial crisis in the NHS that came to a head during the autumn and winter of 1987. Here was a key opportunity for the Government to 'do something about the NHS'.

What they did, however, was not to introduce a Green Paper as suggested by the 1981 departmental review group and which would have inspired an official call for judgements, views, ideas or criticism, but rather a White Paper on NHS reforms, to be published in 1989. And in January 1989, *Working for Patients* (DoH, 1989) was published. During the previous year, the volume of 'evidence' to the review (in fact submitted by proxy to the cross-party House of Commons Social Services Committee) had grown considerably. Perhaps the main topics to be addressed by all who gave their unofficial evidence was that of finance and funding. For most, these were seen as the primary issues, not only because they had come to prominence during the financial crisis in the winter of 1987 (when the Treasury agreed to an emergency cash injection for the NHS of £100 m.) but because they had existed for some time.

A crude summary of the mass of evidence, opinions and alternative reform proposals would place most into three categories: those who believed the NHS to be efficient but underfunded; those who felt it was inefficient, bureaucratic and not underfunded; and lastly those who thought inefficiencies existed but also thought that the NHS could usefully do with some more money.

All who gave evidence led with their ideas on 'the problem with the NHS'. Evidence was usually concluded with 'the answer to the problem with the NHS'. In fact, identifying the 'problem' actually turned out to be quite a difficult exercise. The source of this difficulty was only described by a few, however. For most who gave their views, the problem was that they lacked convincing evidence to support their definition of the problem, and hence their assertion that they had the answer. Arguments were advanced for the privatization (or semi-privatization) of the NHS through the use of subsidized private health-care insurance. This, it was claimed, would deal with the NHS's problem of excessive waiting lists, shabby out-patient waiting rooms, and a number of other ills from which the NHS was commonly held to suffer. Others asserted that lack of money alone was the problem and that with another billion pounds or two (or three, or four . . .) the NHS could get itself back on course to meeting the health-care needs of the population. And there would be no more excessive waiting lists, shabby out-patient waiting rooms, etc.

The uncertainty and anxiety caused by the NHS review tended to encourage people to rush to extremes in many cases. Sometimes these extreme positions were disguised by those giving evidence when they conceded either that – yes – the NHS was good in parts, or that, agreed, it was bad in parts. But the main message in both cases was clear. There was also the suspicion of a tendency for some to play the bargaining/concession game. This consisted in arguing for position A (an extreme position) whilst secretly being satisfied with position B (some compromise between A and C, a position one side suspected the other held).

The real problem, however, is that the information needed to make proper judgements about policy changes in the health field is pathetically slim, missing or just plain confusing. The choices between different policies does not just involve a straightforward comparison of two different states along one quantifiable axis, but, more commonly, decisions involving trade-offs between *many* states and across *many* (more often than not unquantifiable) dimensions. This informational difficulty was not just a problem for those giving evidence to the Government's review, it was also a problem for the authors of the review.

Trials and tribulations

For those who recognized the problem of the lack of information necessary to arrive at sound policies in health care, one answer appeared to be conducting experiments or trials of any major policy changes. Superficially, the reforms of the NHS which were being mooted before the White Paper was published, suggested parallels with the production of a new medical drug whose effects were thought to be beneficial, but on which hard evidence as to the extent of these benefits (and side effects) was lacking. Having invented a new drug, a pharmaceutical company does not have the freedom to sell it merely on the *belief* that it is beneficial; it is obliged to first test the drug's efficacy and safety. This seems straightforwardly sensible. A new health-care system on the other hand, can be freely 'sold' to the public without trial, experiment or test. Whether the public will 'buy' it, of course (or indeed, even have a chance to do so) is another matter.

There were reasons proffered as to why no properly organized trials of the NHS reforms were carried out before embarking on the whole adventure. The Government pointed accusingly at previous reviews and enquiries of the NHS, stating that they would not put up with, as they saw it, the inordinate time these reviews had taken. The Government also pointed out that *Working for Patients* was to take an evolutionary rather than revolutionary approach to change and so exhaustive testing was inappropriate. Mistakes, problems and difficulties were to be sorted out on the job. Ministers at the Department of Health also expressed the view that trials would be used by vested interests to delay and even obstruct any changes the Government wished to introduce. Given that politicians exist to try and change things, then it is understandable that they want to see such changes as they feel are necessary come about. There are, however, technical reasons which make experimentation particularly difficult in the social field. One example illustrates this, taken from the White Paper itself – the internal market or managed competition. How could the concept of splitting purchasers and providers be tested? Would a region be used as a test bed? If so, what happens at the edges, how are inter-regional flows of patients to be dealt with? Trials and tests are also implicit admissions of uncertainty as to outcomes. And if there is one thing a Government – committed to the view that markets are a good thing – would not admit to it is uncertainty over the outcomes of the introduction of a more market-orientated system of running a public-sector industry.

To say that there were no trials of the policies contained in the White Paper is not wholly accurate, however. Some components of the reforms – a collection of somewhat disparate measures and policies – had been around for some time. The resource management initiative, for example, which was to receive a boost from the review of the NHS, had been in existence under one name (clinical budgeting) or another (management budgeting) for many years. The original impetus for resource management was the desire to strengthen the hitherto tenuous connection between that main group in the NHS who are responsible for committing resources at the individual patient level (clinicians), with the wider financial and management responsibility to spend wisely on behalf of all patients. In practice this involved clinicians holding budgets, and this in turn involved a much greater level of accurate and timely cost and activity information.

Improving the monitoring of resource use makes a lot of sense in a health-care system which has integrated the finance and delivery of health care (like the NHS) and which has traditionally been rather poor at knowing exactly the relationship between costs and activity. Aside from the many technical difficulties that have been revealed through experimentation with clinical budgets (providing accurate information to set up and run budgets, for example) it was also found to be difficult to enforce the discipline or accountability that budget holding implies.

Despite the lessons learned from clinical budgeting experiments in the past, the context of resource management has now changed. It may not necessarily be the case that these lessons still apply in a health-care system which has now pulled back a step from its traditional integration of finance and delivery of health care. This contextual problem also affects some of the rather hastily set up 'demonstration districts' or 'locality sites' which concentrated on working through various aspects of the reforms in 1990. The problem with picking on one topic (contracts between purchasers and providers, for instance) was that other aspects of the reforms which were not part of the 'demonstration' (General Practitioner fundholding, for example) are likely to have a significant influence on the outcome of the demonstration. In essence, the White Paper was greater than the sum of its parts.

Almost wholly untested then, health care in the UK has been switched onto a new course. But the changes are not perhaps as radical as some had predicted. The NHS has not been privatized; it is still funded largely from taxation; the private health-care sector has not been encouraged to any significant degree via subsidy or other means to 'take over' the NHS. This does not mean of course that everything has remained the same or that nothing will change over the next ten years.

When it was published, the White Paper was criticized by many for lacking detail. How would the new health-care market actually operate in practice? What guarantees were there to protect patients? How would General Practitioner (GP) budgets work? The lack of detail, the absence of a blueprint, had a lot to do with the sheer speed with which the policies were put together to meet the tight deadline set by the Prime Minister, Mrs Thatcher. Subsequent to its publication however, the White Paper was followed up by numerous 'working papers', Department of Health committees and *ad hoc* demonstration districts and 'action research' projects funded by the Department. The original lack of detail has meant that the broad policy framework set by the White Paper will be implemented over time. In this sense the reforms are 'evolutionary'. Evolution is a powerful process, however, and one which can lead to more radical change than revolution.

THE REFORMS: A SUMMARY

The Government's 'answer to the problem with the NHS' consisted in a range of somewhat disconnected policies and a notable absence of additional funding (at least, additional funding for direct patient care). Some policies represented a continuity of existing changes that were already taking place within the NHS. Others involved the inversion of the objectives of previous changes (for example, the costing systems being developed by the Resource Management Initiative (RMI) were to be used primarily as an aid to billing rather than the intended use, namely, planning). Yet others were new and radical departures from previous economic and managerial structures. Some of the changes required new legislation and this passed through Parliament in 1990 as the NHS and Community Care Act. The changes brought in by the Act ranged from the creation of NHS Trusts to GP budgets and new structures for the membership of health authorities and family practitioner committees. In all, there were around 15 or 16 separate changes, some interdependent, others free-standing.

A brief summary of the changes

- Introduction of weighted capitation to distribute money voted by Parliament for the NHS to Regions and on to Districts.
- Charges for the use and acquisition of capital, including interest and depreciation.
- GP practice budgets for large practices who wished to purchase health care on behalf of their patients.
- In place of the traditional demand-led drug expenditure, 'indicative prescribing "amounts"' (also known as budgets) for GPs to control drug costs and over-prescribing.
- Audit of NHS accounts (including efficiency and effectiveness studies) to be carried out by the independent Audit Commission.
- The separation of the 'providing' and 'purchasing' functions in the NHS; the so-called 'internal market' or 'managed competition'.
- Extension of hospital clinical budgeting (RMI) to over 260 acute units by the end of 1991–92.
- Creation of NHS Trust Hospitals/Units with greater freedom to set pay levels, borrow for capital projects etc. Long-term objective is for all units to become self-governing.
- Changes in the composition of Health Authority and family practitioner committee (FPC) membership. Reduction in numbers; no local authority or trade union representatives.
- Devolved management together with stronger lines of accountability from top to bottom in the NHS.
- FPCs to be made accountable to Regions.
- Consultants' management service to be taken into account in their meritorious service and distinction awards.
- Medical audit to be extended throughout the NHS.
- Consultants' contracts to be more detailed. Managers to be given greater say in contracts.
- A hundred new consultants to be appointed over three years.
- Tax relief on private medical insurance for elderly people.

Not all these reforms have a bearing on the issue of health-care financing, but many do, either directly or indirectly. And sources of finance, how finance is distributed and who it is distributed to, are powerful factors influencing the behaviour of patients, taxpayers, doctors, health service managers and other 'actors' in the health-care game, as well as the sort of health care provided, at what level, and to whom. In arriving at some sort of judgement as to the merits and demerits of any particular financing method, all these factors have to be taken into account. Ultimately, judgements of alternative methods must be based on comparisons of the outcomes different methods produce. These outcomes will include non-medical as well as medical outcomes.

A simple ABC economy

The issue is conceptually very simple: Who pays (A in the above heading)? And how does the money get to the health-care provider (B) in return for treatment and care (C)? If health care were a pair of socks then a reasonably efficient and simple ABC economic system would involve consumers directly purchasing their own socks from a retailer using their own money. Buying socks is usually a straightforward business. The knowledge required by the sock-buying consumer is not too great: foot size, desired colour, material and price are about the only purchasing criteria that are needed – and most can process these variables fairly quickly and without too much trouble so as to make a purchase. Buying socks does not have to be like this. Rather than perusing a few High Street shops, processing the purchasing variables and finally arriving at a decision to buy a pair of black cotton/nylon socks from Marks & Spencer, it is conceivable that a sock agent with specialist knowledge of socks could be consulted. The sock specialist then arranges to 'buy' the socks from the National Hosiery Manufacturers and Distribution Service using the Government issue 'SV' (sock voucher).

Whilst the agent, voucher and nationalized provider system imagined above for socks may seem a nonsensical way of running things, a more or less similar system has been suggested as a way of providing and distributing health care in this country. The point, however, is that there are many different ways of organizing the basic ABC economy, whether it is for socks or health care. It is not always obvious, however, that one way is better (however that is defined) than another.

Ruling out the obviously bizarre or plainly ludicrous ways of financing health care, there are in essence only four basic alternative methods:

1 Direct payment by users
2 Private health insurance

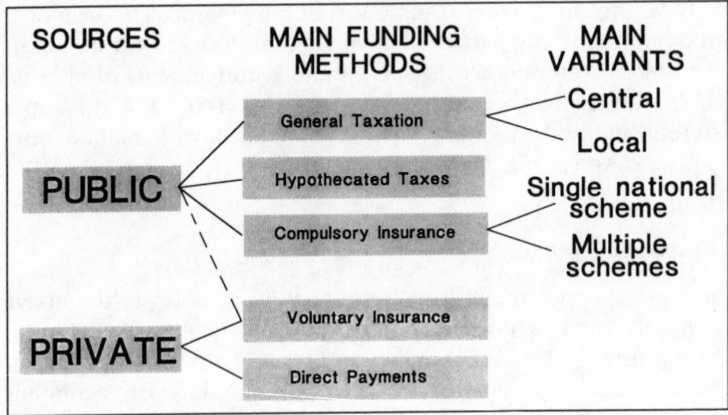

Figure 1.1 Alternatives for health-care financing.
Source: Maxwell (1988).

3 Social or state insurance
4 Direct tax

Within each basic method, as Maxwell *et al.* (1988b) have noted, there are many variants, and there are many combinations of basic methods (and their variants) possible within one health-care system (see Figure 1.1). Moreover, there are many ways of completing the transaction involving A and B in return for C within each financing method. All health-care systems are pluralistic with respect to financing (and organization) with tendencies to one method rather than another. Health care in the UK is currently a combination of methods, (1), (2) and (4) with additions such as charitable funding, lotteries, income generation and land and estate sales. Health care in the UK tends towards (4).

International comparisons

In other countries they do things differently. Tables 1.1 and 1.2 illustrate the variations in public/private funding and sources of funding respectively. The German health-care system tends towards method (3) (with varying proportions of the other basic methods). In the USA, the health-care economy is dominated by private health insurance but with a significant proportion of

Table 1.1 Public/private financing split (1987): selected international comparisons

Country	*Percentage of total health care financing from:*	
	Public sector	*Private sector*
Norway	97.6	2.4
Luxembourg	91.6	8.4
Sweden	90.8	9.2
Iceland	88.5	11.5
Ireland	87.0	13.0
UK	86.4	13.6
Denmark	85.5	14.5
New Zealand	82.5	17.5
Italy	79.2	20.8
Finland	78.6	21.4
Germany	78.4	21.6
Belgium	76.9	23.1
Greece	75.2	24.8
France	74.8	25.2
Canada	73.9	26.1
Netherlands	73.9	26.1
Japan	73.0	27.0
Spain	71.5	28.5
Australia	70.5	29.5
Switzerland	68.2	31.8
Austria	67.1	32.9
Portugal	60.7	39.3
USA	41.4	58.6
Turkey	41.3	58.7

Source: OECD (1989)

government-funded (i.e. direct tax) care. In Switzerland, 25 per cent of total health-care expenditure comes from social insurance, 33 per cent from direct payments and 40 per cent from general taxes. The Swedish system looks more like that of the UK's in financing terms, with the greatest proportion of funding (80 per cent) coming from general taxes and only small amounts from social insurance and direct payments. Private insurance is virtually non-existent in Sweden. The French tend towards social insurance

Table 1.2 Sources of finance (1975): selected international comparisons (in percentages)

Country	*General taxation*	*Social insurance*	*Direct payments*	*Private insurance*
UK	87.3	5.0	5.8	1.2
Sweden	78.5	13.1	8.4	–
Switzerland	41.7	24.8	33.5	–
USA	31.1	11.7	27.1	25.6
Germany	14.6	62.5	12.5	5.3
France	7.0	69.0	19.6	3.0

Source: Maxwell (1981)

(70 per cent of health-care expenditure) and direct payments (20 per cent of expenditure). Less than 10 per cent of general taxation is spent on health care. And so on around the globe.

Different countries with various combinations and permutations of financing methods apply them in different ways. Sometimes different financing methods are associated with specific forms of health care. In the UK, acupuncture, for example, is not financed by direct taxes but is instead purchased directly by users from private acupuncturists. In the USA, the state-funded insurance programmes of Medicaid and Medicare are linked to particular groups of the population (low-income families and elderly people, respectively). These two programmes account for around 30 per cent of total health-care spending in the USA.

The plethora of different forms of health-care systems around the world with their different ways of financing and organizing the basic transaction between A and B in exchange for C seems to imply that there is no single, unique or right way of doing things when it comes to health care. It could also mean that different health-care systems have evolved to suit different societies with different ideas and notions of medicine or the citizen's right to care, for example. (It is worth noting in passing that factors such as chance, blunder, mistake, history, accident and happenstance should not be underestimated when it comes to explanations as to why particular health-care systems are as they are.) But health-care systems are continually evolving and changing, and it could be that, cultural differences and traditions aside, there will be some convergence in the way different countries organize and finance their respective systems. This last interpretation suggests perhaps that progress in the way health-care systems are financed and organized is like time's arrow – never going backwards but always moving forwards. This is not necessarily the case.

NON-NEUTRALITY OF FINANCING SYSTEMS

There would appear to be many ways of running the ABC economy of health care. And perhaps there is a perfect way of doing so. One 'perfect' way is implied by a line from an essay in the Centre for Policy Studies' *The Litmus Papers* (Cozens-Hardy, 1980), 'What does it matter where the money comes from [for health care] as long as it comes?' This begs the question of course. As long as there is enough money to satisfy all needs, then there would be no need for economists, or politicians, or any of the other dismal professions who struggle with the seemingly intractable problem of making, or helping to make, choices. As there are not enough resources to do everything human beings want/need/desire to do there is a basic need to make choices. But moreover, even if the economist's argument of finite resources/infinite demand is accepted, it does matter where the money comes from to pay for health care. Not least it matters to those who pay. But more than this, experience shows that different sources of funding can directly influence the *way* health care is provided, *how* much is provided, *who* provides it, *what* is provided and to *whom* it is provided.

He who pays the piper

The state-run health-care insurance scheme in the USA for low-income families, Medicaid, is funded from state and federal general taxes. The nature of Medicaid funding gives the state the power to control how these funds are used. In the case of Medicaid they are specifically directed to low-income families to help plug one of the major gaps in health-care coverage which the private insurance market failed to do. A further example comes from the UK where the funding of the NHS primarily from general taxation has given government a central role in determining health-care priorities as well as placing the NHS firmly in the public political arena and hence subject to competing priorities between spending departments.

Equity

There is another reason why the source and method of health-care financing cannot assume to be neutral or of no material importance when it comes to the source of funding for health care. This concerns an almost universally recognized goal in health care, namely, equity or a notion of 'fairness'. One interpretation of this notion of fairness suggests that we, the users of health care, want more than just successful treatment for ourselves when we are ill; we also want others to have successful treatment when they are ill. This may be pure altruism or it may be a combination of altruism and self-interest ('I would like people with infectious diseases not to be restricted in their access to treatment because they may infect me', for example). There are many other possible interpretations of what is meant by 'fairness' – equality of access to health care? Equality of outcome of health-care intervention? Equal treatment for equal need? However the concept is defined, there is a consensual feeling that equity in the health-care field should be important. So how can the source of funding for health care affect equity?

It is not possible to prove the existence of a relationship between systems of funding and equity without reference to empirical evidence. However, the evidence tends to support the intuitive belief that funding health care from, say, progressive taxes levied on those in work is more equitable than a system which treats health care as just another commodity to be bought if it can be afforded. Even if the level of illness (and hence the amount of health-care resources needed to deal with it) were spread evenly across all income groups, direct payment for health care would, on balance, leave the poor worse off than the rich. Not only that, but some of the poor are likely to be so poor that they cannot afford to buy health care in the first place. It should be noted in passing that 'poor' is a relative concept. With a hip operation in the NHS currently costing around £3000 and one year's worth of the anti-anaemia drug for renal failure patients – erythropoietin – costing about £5000, you do not have to be particularly 'poor' to find payment difficult.

In a country where health care is funded solely from a progressive tax system (and with health care provided free at the time of need – otherwise the system in essence reverts to one funded by direct payments, albeit in a rather roundabout way) the situation tends to be more equitable. How equity is to be defined and then how it is to be measured are other questions which, as with the basic correlative proof of the relationship between funding and equity, requires hard data on, for example, contributions to the health-care system and benefits received by different groups in the population.

SUMMARY

For those in the UK born after 1948 there has effectively been only one kind of health-care system, the NHS. Throughout the nineteenth century, public provision of health care was mainly limited to the Poor Law's boards of guardians, who offered free services to those who could pass a means test. In 1911 the medical provisions of the Insurance Act provided for limited medical coverage to limited sections of the population. The unemployed and dependants of those in employment were not covered by the Act. The middle and upper classes were also not covered. In the main, the only hospital care offered under National Health Insurance (NHI) was for tuberculosis sufferers. Between the means-tested service of the Poor Law and direct payment for services offered by private medical practitioners stood the poorly equipped and fragmented medical care provided by charitable hospitals and some local authorities. For most of the population it was not only the occurrence of ill health which was uncertain, but the means by which good health could be secured through medical treatment and care. The advent of the NHS for the first time comprehensively tackled that latter uncertainty and in so doing began to tackle the former uncertainty.

Now, in the 1990s, and after over 40 years of an overwhelmingly public health service funded from general taxation and provided free to those in need at the time of use, the NHS is starting to embark on a new and uncertain course. Its dominance on the supply side is likely to be increasingly challenged by the private sector, perhaps accelerating a trend begun in the early 1980s. As private health-care insurance companies perhaps take encouragement from provisions arising from the reforms of the NHS and start to expand the scope and coverage of their policies, the balance of total health-care funding is likely to change. The new competitive framework set in place by the reforms contains, necessarily, at its heart an uncertainty for the NHS. Competition, albeit on the limited scale and with the regulatory rules currently in place, will possibly lead to considerable restructuring of health-care provision in the UK. On the one hand, the potential failure of the current reforms to deliver politically could lead to renewed pressure to take the reforms further and perhaps to question the very basis of funding of health care directly. On the other hand, the reforms, like supertankers, could build up a considerable momentum of their own, again with potentially far reaching implications for the financing of health care.

Aside from the internal forces for change embodied in the NHS reforms, there are external forces perhaps even more powerful which will undoubtedly ensure some degree of change in the way health care is funded and provided: changes in the population (its size and structure), changes in the nation's wealth (recession or boom?), changes in medical ideas, opportunities and discoveries (domiciliary not hospital care, gene therapy), changes in medical priorities (AIDS), changes in government priorities and changes in government itself. All these factors and many more will exert pressures, to a lesser or greater extent, on health services over the coming decade. The pressure on health-care finances is likely to be very great indeed and the economy of health care will be redirected in any of a number of ways. This does not mean that its eventual destination is inevitable, however. Along the route there will be many chances to exercise some choice as to the way health care is paid for, in what way and by whom. It may be the case that we get the politicians (the professional choice-makers) we deserve, but it is essential that we get the health-care system of our choice. Before making that choice, however, it is wise to consider the possible outcomes different choices imply; for what we may want is not necessarily what we may need.

Financing health care in the 1990s

The remaining chapters of this book examine some of the issues concerning the financing of health care, in particular, but not exclusively, arising from the new direction the NHS is now embarked upon. In general, the book follows a course starting at some of the financial issues raised by the reforms and ending up with some views of the future in terms of the financing of health care in the UK. On route, particular topics are examined, from the way health care has been financed in the past, to some of the arguments which have been put forward concerning the level of health-care financing, and examples of different systems of financing and funding.

In particular, Chapter 2 looks at the recent reforms of the NHS and the possible ramifications these changes have for health-care financing. Chapter 3 traces the history of public and private financing of health care back to 1948 and identifies trends which could be important in understanding the future. The history of public health-care financing has been dogged since the inception of the NHS by one particular issue, the level of funding. This will be one criterion against which not only the recent reforms will be (at least popularly) judged, but also any alternative way of financing or organizing health care in the UK. In Chapter 4, alternative ideas concerning how the level of health-care funding could be determined are examined. Chapters 5, 6 and 7 describe three methods of financing health care, from direct payment and private insurance through to various refinements and variants of the basic insurance method (health maintenance organizations, preferred provider organizations, state or social insurance). These chapters draw on the experience of health-care systems in other countries – in particular the USA and Germany – to describe a move along a continuum from free to regulated market. Financing options are complicated as the permutations and combinations possible are almost endless. However, for the time being many options seem unlikely given current policies and directions. Nevertheless, as the 1990s progress, the reforms of the NHS are likely to lead health care into unexpected regions. External factors will also shape the UK's health-care system, the way it is organized, the way it is structured, the balance between public and private sectors, the services provided and also the way it is funded and financed. Chapter 8 picks up and develops the issues identified in Chapter 2 to provide possible scenarios of the way health care may be financed over the coming decade.

Chapter 9 draws together some of the main themes concerning health-care financing. It is clear that there are no easy answers to the question of how to finance health care; the ideal system does not exist, even if we knew and could agree how to define what is meant by ideal. This does not mean that the way health care is financed cannot be improved, but in doing so there are likely to be difficult decisions to be taken and trade-offs to be made.

2

SEEDS OF CHANGE

Despite the billions of words and the millions of person-hours devoted to the reforms of the NHS there still remains a distinct aura of uncertainty about the future. But should there be? This chapter explores some particular aspects of the NHS reforms which, either directly or indirectly, appear to contain the seeds of potentially quite radical change in the UK's health-care economy.

THE REFORM'S INTENTIONS: OPAQUE OR TRANSPARENT?

In its concluding remarks, a commentary from the Nuffield Institute for Health Service Studies (1989) noted:

> This latest set of reforms stands apart from the others in its opacity and imprecision. Whether intentional or not, it confounds any attempt to predict the outcome with any certainty at all.

Such remarks were typical of many reviews of the Review. But were these reforms really 'opaque' in the sense that one could not see through them either to some ultimate outcome or, at the very least, to the intended objective? The reforms certainly appeared at first sight to be a rather mixed bag of changes. But there are a number of policy changes which, from the point of view of the financing of health care, not only fit together in a reasonably logical way, but, it can be argued, make up a definite policy shift in health care, namely, the introduction of a more pluralistic health-care economy, with a greater mix of finance sources and a greater variety of health-care providers. Even if this were not the intended outcome (and it is not how the White Paper itself sums up the reforms), it is a very likely outcome given the policy seeds that have been sown by the reforms. Given the many reforms by the current Government in other areas of the public sector, for example, its explicit macroeconomic policies, decentralization in education and local government, its general philosophy of the role of government in public life and, importantly, the particular belief in a personal freedom of choice based on the individual's inalienable right to dispose of their post-tax income as they see fit, it is not difficult to argue that it is virtually axiomatic that pluralism, mix and variety in health care are the intentional outcomes of the reforms.

Furthermore, is it also really the case that the reforms were that imprecise? Or, put another way, was it actually necessary to be that precise given the intended outcome identified above? Whilst it is true that on certain specifics the reforms did lack the necessary detail for implementation, it could be argued that one of the central changes, the separation of the purchasing and providing roles in health care, did not actually require that much elaboration or detail; a market is a market, and one particular characteristic of markets is their freedom to set their own rules, find their own equilibrium and do business in their own way. There was, at least from the Government's point of view, no need to describe in detail how this new market in health care would operate. Although the White Paper studiously avoided any mention of the word 'market', its policies cannot be interpreted as anything else except as, at the minimum, market-orientated.

Just prior to the publication of the White Paper, two schools of thought developed concerning the changes the White Paper would advocate. The first was essentially the belief that the policy changes would effectively sum to nothing, that in the end the combination of the power of the medical profession and other interested parties, as well as the seemingly enormous political hurdle of the popularity of the NHS (despite all its shortcomings), would just prove too insurmountable and in the end too risky politically for effective and radical change to be introduced. The other school contended that, on its past record, the Government would not shrink from grasping the nettle, and that the NHS was in for some momentous change. In this chapter it is argued that, in fact, both schools were right – it is just the timing of their predictions that was wrong. From a slow start, the reforms have the potential for considerable change in the way health care is financed in the UK.

As with much of the unofficial evidence to the Government's behind-closed-doors review, *Working for Patients* identified what it thought was 'the problem with the NHS'. These included such things as apparently inexplicable variations in performance between Health Authorities in terms of, for example, the cost of treatment per patient, variations in GP referral rates and a lack of 'consumer' responsiveness. The Government's diagnosis was, as the Nuffield Institute (1989) pointed out, rather narrow, omitting the whole issue of persistent health inequalities, the level of preventable illness and the widespread allegation that the NHS was underfunded. The omission of this latter aspect is perhaps not surprising given the Government's robust defence of its level of funding of the NHS since 1980. Whilst most commentators would agree that it was the financial crisis in the cash-limited hospital and community health services wing of the NHS in 1987 which spurred the Government's review of 1988 and eventual reforms of 1989, it cannot be overlooked that the 1987 crisis provided a prime political opportunity to whip off the dust covers from previous internal reviews of the NHS and present them at a time of general criticism of the NHS and, indeed, of the Government's policies towards the NHS.

BUT NOTHING HAS CHANGED

Apart from the notable lack of any concessions to those who argued before, during and after the publication of *Working for Patients* that the underlying problem with the NHS was underfunding, the other absence of note was the lack of any apparent change in the source of funding for the NHS. The NHS is still to be funded largely from general taxation (78.3 per cent in 1989–90) with additions coming from NHS contributions (16.2 per cent) and patients' payments such as prescription charges, plus miscellaneous income (5.5 per cent). There has been no introduction of compulsory private or public medical insurance. Vouchers have not been printed and distributed for the public to exchange for the health care of their choice. No new hypothecated (earmarked) tax has been invented specifically to finance the NHS. And there has been no introduction of alternative financing methods from the overtly inequitable end of the tax spectrum such as a flat-rate community charge.

So, nothing has changed. Or has it? There are a number of specific policy changes which have the potential (and, it might be assumed, the intention) to alter the way health care is financed over the next ten years, all things being equal. The first, and perhaps the most important, is the separation of two responsibilities in health care – provision (supply) and purchase (demand). The parenthetical words are there to jog the parallel, which is, of course, with the notion of a market.

The separation of purchasers and providers

No longer do health authorities manage the services provided by the hospital and community units within (and occasionally outside) their borders. Instead health authorities have a new role, to assess the health needs of their resident population and then to purchase health-care services to meet that assessed need up to the constraint of the allocation they have been given by their Regional Health Authorities. But here lies the central point, for there will not be just one purchaser (the District Health Authority) but many, from private individuals to medical insurance companies and the private health-care sector. This variety of purchasers suggests a variety of financing sources and methods. Of these new purchasers, it is the medical-insurance sector purchasing health care on behalf of their subscribers which is likely to grow the fastest.

NHS Trusts: new incentives?

It is the introduction of NHS Trusts on the supply side of this new health-care market, which will spur the business imperative and encourage new purchasers and hence new sources and methods of financing health care. The use of the word 'hospital' is a slight misnomer as a Trust could include anything from a small acute hospital, to an amalgam of acute and community units and onwards to the entire services previously supplied by a District Health Authority or, indeed, an ambulance service. The move to NHS Trusts is to be gradual, without any coercion (overtly, at least). The 'first wave' candidates in 1991 numbered 57 (of – as has been noted – all varieties). And the stated intention of the Government is for all units to eventually become Trusts. Units which have not become Trusts occupy the halfway house of directly managed status; managed, that is, by their current District Health Authorities.

Although this management is supposed to be carried out at arm's length, in reality District Health Authorities are likely to find it difficult to withdraw completely from the management of their units, at least in the short term. Trusts, on the other hand, are different.

Whilst technically still part of the NHS, with Boards accountable to the Secretary of State, their ethos is independence, not the dependence of the directly managed unit (DMU). The outlook of the Trust is the outlook of a business. With no guaranteed income (but with enhanced freedoms to, for example, borrow money and set pay and conditions of service) the overriding incentive (or business imperative) is to search for and encourage custom, not just from Health Authorities, but from other purchasers of health care. In this sense the formation of Trusts serves to bolster the potential changes in the balance of health-care finance, arising as a result of the separation of purchasers and providers. In particular, given that one group of purchasers (Districts) will be strictly cash-limited, Trusts are likely to seek out alternative income sources. One significant source will be the private health-care/insurance sector.

Tax relief on private medical insurance

A further policy change to note is one that has been a little overlooked since its introduction but which is perhaps one of the most important changes to arise out of the review of the NHS in terms of the precedent it sets. From April 1990, elderly people (that is, those aged over 60) with a taxable income, or those who pay their premiums, have been able to claim tax relief on their medical insurance premium payments. Whilst in the short term this tax relief (which can also be seen as a potential subsidy to private health care) is unlikely to induce any significant increase in the number of this age group holding private medical insurance, its price-reducing effect, coupled with the implied encouragement to private medical insurers to develop more appealing policies with wider coverage available to more people, has the possibility to alter the balance of total health-care funding in the longer run. Moreover, because it sets a precedent, there is room to speculate about its extension to other age, social or work groups.

Alternative sources of income

In addition to these specific policy changes, there is a set of changes which, whilst they are not new, receive an impetus because of the reforms of the NHS and which have the potential to change, if not the very nature of health-care finance, at least its balance.

Whilst health care remains, naturally enough, the main line of business, the extra freedoms given to providers (and in particular, to Trusts) coupled with the exigencies of the enforced separation of providers from a guaranteed source of income, means that generation of income, of whatever sort and from whatever source, is likely to grow in significance. Although in-store hospitals are an unlikely development, in-hospital stores are not. And although 'vertical integration' into the undertaking business is not something even the keenest Trust business manager with a profit motive and a gloomy financial forecast in their hands is likely to suggest to their Board, vertical integration the other way, into the marketing of, for example, specially developed medical equipment or pharmaceuticals, is not unimaginable. Indeed, it is to some extent already happening now.

Non-health-care income generation may provide additional cash over and above that raised by taxation and allocated to the health service. On the other hand, this extra income may be offset at national level by the Treasury when it negotiates with the Department of Health each year over the NHS budget (that is, District Health Authorities' purchasing incomes) in the same way that it has tended to do with the NHS's internally generated efficiency savings (the cost improvement programme). Furthermore, the deregulation ethos of the NHS reforms may lead to the full privatization of some services such as occurred with the privatization of eye tests.

CHANGES IN THE FIRST YEAR

The first year of the Government's reforms, 1991, has been, by and large, a confirmation of the 'no real change' school of thought. Stability has been the keyword. The separation of District Health Authorities from their responsibilities for hands-on management of the people, buildings and equipment necessary to provide health care has occurred. Hospital and community units have parted company with their budgets. Bridging the gap between these halves of the purchaser/provider divide are thousands of contracts setting out the services health authorities want units to provide and the price they are going to pay. Whilst mergers of a sort have taken place on the provider side – some districts' entire services having become Trusts – no units have been liquidated, patients flow where they always have, by and large, flowed and units have received an income via their contracts more or less equivalent to the previous year's allocated budget. The first year was not without some noticeable events, however. Plans by some Trusts (and DMUs) to cut costs by reducing staff numbers and cutting back on some services in order to become more competitive, were not predicted to occur – at least, not yet.

However, in general, there has been continuity with pre-reformation days through a combination of price-fixing and direct intervention by Regions and the Government. This continuity has also been maintained by ignorance – ignorance on the part of purchasing Districts as to the real health needs of their populations and of the alternatives to long-standing service patterns, for example. But it is also hard to change existing patterns of service because start-up and entry costs are so high in health care: new hospitals take time to be built and existing acute hospitals (in the NHS at least) have generally operated at 80–90 per cent occupancy, so altering patient referrals will require extensions and additions, which again take time.

Stability is, therefore, hardly surprising. Especially so, considering the introduction of important changes in the way the total health service budget is shared out amongst Regions and Districts. The introduction of managed competition and Districts' responsibilities for their own residents' health-care needs (rather than the needs of patients, resident and non-resident, treated by their units) necessitated a transformation in the old way of sharing out the health budget. Over the next few years the allocative system will be moving towards one based mainly on the size and age structure of their resident population (with additions or subtractions to equate for differences in mortality levels between districts). This weighted capitation will mean that many Districts have received substantially altered allocations compared with 1990–91. The first, transitional, year began the move to full weighted capitation. Without this gradualist approach, disruption to hospital and community services could have been considerable.

CHANGES IN SUBSEQUENT YEARS

It was perhaps inevitable that the first year of the reforms would see little change. This is not to underestimate the massive cultural change that the NHS has undergone, not just in this first year, but in the years since the publication of *Working for Patients*. Nor is it to underestimate the considerable managerial change (not to mention effort and time) that has happened or the vastly accelerated pace of change of initiatives such as resource management with all the information implications that entails. The point is that both politically and practically, change could not be allowed to happen too quickly.

But what of the future? Are existing referral patterns still to be followed? Is the health service to remain paralysed, not deviating from its 1991-set course? This is a possibility, but it seems very unlikely and a total negation of all the reforms. What seems much more likely is that the various actors in the health-care game start to learn how to play by the new rules. From patients (and potential patients) to central government, NHS Trusts, District Health Authorities, GP fund holders, private hospitals, medical insurance companies and back to clinicians, health-care workers and managers, all will be involved in the new health-care market. The game they will be learning to play had its rules specified in the reforms of 1989–90. And these rules were set, as has already been intimated, so as to encourage a more pluralistic health-care system in the UK, with a greater variety of health-care providers and a greater mix of financing sources and methods. This is a direct echo of the internal Department of Health ministerial advice paper from 1981 and quoted in Chapter 1.

So what are the implications for health-care financing? Already outlined are a number of policy changes arising from the reforms which have the potential to alter the balance and method of health-care financing in the UK. In addition, there is a clutch of pre-reformation trends in financing which are likely to receive a boost either from specific policy changes or from the general thrust of the reforms. Before examining these issues in more detail, it is worth noting just one of the factors which will inevitably blur the image of this crystal-ball gazing exercise.

Problems with predictions

Two things can go wrong with predictions, no matter how firmly based or apparently obvious they seem to be at the time. The first is that the things predicted to happen just do not happen at all. The second is that the predictions are partly correct, but the size of the predicted changes is wrong. The sheer number and complexity of interaction of the prediction-confounding variables in health care should be warning enough not to contemplate even the most highly qualified and hedged prediction of what is likely to be even one year from now, let alone two to ten years from now.

After attempting to describe mathematically the ten-dimensional motion of a bicycle, Stewart (1990), a specialist in the highly complex field of the mathematics of chaos, observed that economists make predictions about systems which occupy spaces of thousands of dimensions. So, economists work in a sort of *n*-dimensional hyperspace and non-economists wonder why economists are always disagreeing with each other and getting their forecasts wrong. Out of the thousands of factors (dimensions) which lie in wait for the puny three-dimensional economist, one of the most confounding is politics. Or, more precisely, a change of government. With a change of government can come a significant change in policy. And it can be guaranteed that health care, being firmly embedded in the political milieu, will not escape the ineluctable urge of politicians to leave their mark.

The only way out of this difficulty is either to know what future governments have in mind for changes in policy (and it is not at all clear that even future governments know what they have in mind) or, in essence, to ignore the problem. The intention here is to take the latter course as the purpose of this chapter is to try and examine some of the limits of trends in current and recent health-care policy changes rather than speculate about as yet inarticulated and certainly unimplemented policy changes in the future.

Market opportunities, market imperatives

The separation of the functions of health-care purchase and provision represents one of the most important changes introduced by the NHS reforms, for it is the first necessary (but not sufficient) step towards the creation of a market in health care. It can be argued that what now exists (and what will exist) is not a market that any private sector firm would recognize, that it is 'managed competition', a controlled and highly regulated market. Health authorities may have boards of directors but there are no share holders; interest and depreciation is now paid by the health service for the use of capital just like private-sector firms, but only Trusts have (limited) freedoms to borrow from the commercial sector. It may be controlled, managed and regulated, but then so are many, if not all, markets. What is important as far as the issue of financing health care (and, of course, other aspects of health care) is concerned is how the actors interpret, use and are influenced by, the new rules and regulations, the freedoms, the incentives and the disincentives in this new set up.

On the purchasing side in this new health-care system what is interesting is that health authorities are just one (admittedly the biggest) purchaser amongst many. Alongside health authorities there are now GP fund holders and local authorities. Increasingly, however, private medical insurers, private-sector health-care providers (in their purchasing role buying particular services from NHS directly-managed hospitals and Trusts) and private individuals buying health-care directly, are likely to increase their profile in this system. To borrow a term from the field of international relations, one of the consequences of the NHS reforms is to break the *hegemony* of the health authority as health-care financier.

The reduction in the financial power and influence of the health authority will arise for a number of reasons, all working in concert. The first, and not to be underestimated, is to do with a cultural shift which has been induced by the reforms. The megalith of the NHS has been fragmented by the separation of the purchasing and providing roles; new purchasers (primarily the private medical insurers on behalf of their subscribers and particularly GPs with budgets) now have a clearer view of, and access to, NHS providers. There is a strong likelihood of a rising trend in private medical-insurance policyholders (potentially receiving a boost from a continuing restraint in public health-care financing) as a result of this new openness and the financial incentives facing GP budget holders. The fragmentation of the NHS looks set to give rise to a new balance in health-care financing, as the pluralistic objective of the reforms is realized.

Of these various factors, perhaps the most important is the prospects for continued growth in the private medical-insurance market (it would perhaps be better to drop the word 'private' as health-care providers will increasingly include the NHS). The most pertinent factor here is the cost of medical insurance (especially as for most people there is no offsetting reduction in tax). Although medical insurance premiums have risen considerably over the last few years, recent moves by general insurance companies (e.g.

Norwich Union, Abbey Life, Eagle Star, etc.) suggest that the competition in the medical-insurance market will increase. Indeed, the health-care manager for London & Edinburgh Insurance has predicted that the provident associations' share of the insurance market is likely to fall from its current dominant 90 per cent to 75 per cent over the next ten years (*Health Service Journal*, 1990). Such competition is more than likely to reduce medical insurance premiums – at least in the short run. But even if the costs of insurance reduce, is this enough of an incentive on its own for people to take up insurance?

What seems to unite the confusing evidence on the reasons some people go private is the overriding belief that they are getting something more than they would if they were simply an NHS patient. And it is exactly this 'something more' that Trusts, those new business-orientated health-care providers created by the 1990 NHS Act, are likely to want to provide to private patients as the hospitals tap every available market for their services. Trusts (and it should be remembered that the plan is for all NHS units to eventually become Trusts) would not be acting sensibly if they did not look to increase income from the private insurance sector, when faced with a major purchaser (the District Health Authority) who is unlikely to see their purchasing power increase in line with demand judging from past experience.

Indeed, given its previous record, this major purchaser may have difficulty increasing their purchasing power in line with inflation, let alone demand. Following on from this, it seems unlikely, therefore, that NHS patients (whose care is purchased on their behalf by cash-limited health authorities) will see the sort of improvements in the way their care is provided (no waiting lists, pre-arranged admission, choice of doctor, etc.) that would perhaps prevent an increasing number of people turning to private medical insurance; the 'negative' image of the NHS is reinforced for those contemplating 'going private'. Ironically perhaps, whilst the source of funding may be increasingly private, the provision of care could increasingly be public, as Trusts move into private provision in order to diversify and at the same time protect their income.

So, on the one side there are Trusts facing the incentive to search out and promote alternative sources of income, and on the other there are potential customers with, as they see it, an incentive to opt for private financing of their health-care needs.

Subsidizing private medical insurance

Tax relief for private medical-insurance policies for people aged over 60 years was introduced in April 1990. Up to now, however, it does not appear to have had a significant impact on the take up of insurance. This is not to say that this tax break will not encourage higher take up in the future, or that because it has so far had a negligible effect on the number of this age group holding medical insurance, the policy itself is not important or significant. In some ways, its apparent failure may be a spur to greater lobbying pressure on the Government to make it work, to make it achieve its underlying aim of increasing the number of private medical-insurance policyholders. Laing (1990) has argued that from the perspective of the insurance and private health-care provider industries there is scope for lobbying to relax some of the qualifying restrictions on the 1990 scheme. Furthermore, tax relief may encourage insurers to devise more appropriate and attractive policies for the elderly.

As with the stimulus to the medical-insurance market resulting from the separation of providers and purchasers and the setting up of Trusts, tax breaks for medical insurance for people aged over 60 years has the potential, the seeds, to change the balance of health-care financing in the UK.

Generating income

For the NHS, income generation has, since 1 April 1991, taken on a new significance. Income generation is not now the sidelines of florist shops or charging for car parks; it includes the generation of income from selling health care. But whilst income from selling health-care services is – and will remain – the main source of revenue for health-care providers, the 'sidelines' are likely to increase in importance.

A survey by the National Association of Health Authorities and Trusts (NAHAT, 1990a) showed that income generation schemes by Health Authorities in England, Wales and Northern Ireland were raising £70 m. in recurring income with a further £20 m. in new income in 1990–91. In one sense these sums are small; only amounting to about 0.6 per cent of health authorities' total revenue budget in 1990–91. But £90 m. is £90 m., and each year since 1984 (when the Government began to actively encourage the NHS to engage in income-generation schemes) the sums have got larger. Left to their own devices it seems unlikely, however, that Health Authorities would ever come to rely too heavily on non-health-care-generated income. But Health Authorities have not been left to their own devices, and the newly created providers now have some strong financial incentives to search out *any* income opportunity. This does not mean that hospitals will suddenly decide to move into the banking or retail food business. But, in looking at their resources, in particular the often quite unique knowledge, skills and specialized equipment they have access to or own, health-care providers may find themselves very well placed to exploit other health-care related markets. Pharmaceuticals, medical equipment, catering, pathology services are all examples of areas where expertise has been concentrated in the NHS.

CONCLUSION

This chapter has explored some of the possible financing ramifications of the Government's reforms of the NHS. It has suggested that far from being vague and imprecise, the reforms contain a certain logic and structure with regard to the financing of health care which is likely to lead to more pluralism in financing.

For the third largest organization in the world, significant change is obviously difficult to bring about; the NHS has a high inertia factor. Moreover, deviation from previous patterns of provision and financing in the first year of the reforms have been heavily proscribed; evolutionary, not disruptive change was the desired option. Nevertheless, the reforms of the Service begun in 1988, have great potential to bring about realignments in the source of health-care financing over the next ten years. Perhaps the greatest change has been in its economic environment. The separation of the purchasing and providing roles, the creation of a pseudo-market in health care, the creation of NHS Trusts, the introduction of new and different incentives in management and a more overt linking of the financing of care with the provision of care, all tend to suggest that the method of financing will not remain static.

3

PAST TRENDS IN HEALTH-CARE FUNDING

Chapter 2 highlighted a number of issues arising from the reforms of the NHS as they might affect the future of health-care financing in the UK. There is, however, another way of looking at the future and that is by looking at the past. What have been the post-war patterns of UK health-care expenditure and financing? And to what extent do these provide indications for future trends?

THE RISE AND RISE OF THE NHS

Even the most cursory glance of the health-care spending figures in the period since 1948 reveals the overwhelming dominance of the public sector in the finance of health care in the UK. For example, spending on the NHS has accounted for between 85 and 90 per cent of total health-care spending. What the figures also show is the quite enormous increase in the amount of money spent on the NHS every year since the war (see, for example, Figure 3.1).

It was as early as December 1948 – just five months after the inception of the Service – that the future pattern for NHS spending was set. On 13 December 1948 Aneurin Bevan had to tell the Cabinet that the estimate for the first nine months' NHS expenditure of £176 m. was some £50 m. short. As Campbell (1987) has pointed out in his biography of Bevan, one week into the new Service and it became apparent that a miscalculation had been made 'so fundamental that it virtually negated the central assumption on which the Service had been set up'. The miscalculation was, of course, how much the NHS would actually cost to run. Not only had the Ministry of Health simply projected forward estimates of

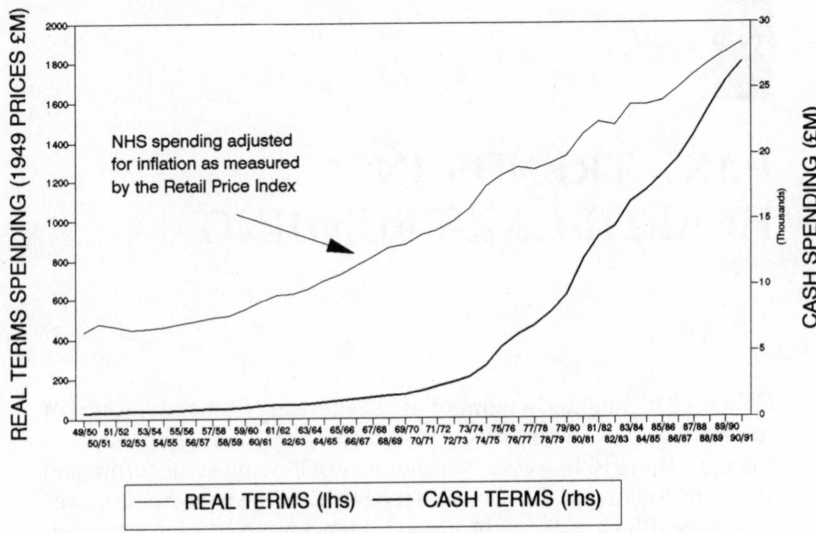

Figure 3.1 Total UK NHS expenditure: cash and real spending.

Sources: OHE (1990); DoH (1991).

pre-war health-care spending, the health-care planners and politicians of the day had assumed that, as the population benefited from the new Service, and consequently became healthier, that spending would actually decline.

With the benefit of over 40 years' hindsight this assumption appears highly unrealistic. Indeed, the evidence of miscalculation arose almost immediately the Service started. The rush for spectacles and dental treatment was overwhelming and immediate. In the first full year, over 8 million people – 16 per cent of the population – were seeking dental treatment. Similar numbers also made use of the free ophthalmic service. In the first few months of the NHS, over 95 per cent of the population had signed up to GPs. And the numbers of doctors, dentists, chemists and opticians who joined the fledgling Service was over 47 000. Bevan himself admitted that with the feeling that everything was now free it somehow did not matter what was charged to the Exchequer. But this economic textbook example of the effects of zero-pricing should not overshadow the fact that there was real need for the services and treatments offered by the NHS. The previously 'hidden' demand for health care was now uncovered.

There were other problems and issues at the beginning: apart from Bevan's generous financial inducements to doctors to take part in the new service, miscalculations of dentists' fees leading to overpayment and large rises in the pay of other medical staff (accounting for two-thirds of the entire budget in the first year) contributed to the Ministry's spending miscalculations. A further reason for the Ministry's underestimates was suggested by Honigsbaum (1989). It was not so much a question of miscalculation, but of self-imposed restraint: the Ministry felt the Treasury would not give them the money they needed, so they opted instead for an acceptably modest but insufficient level of funding.

Bevan's main argument during a Parliamentary debate over the extra £50 m. he claimed the NHS needed in its first year was essentially that the NHS was a victim of its own success; its success in attracting medical and other health-care workers to join the Service and its success in attracting patients in their millions. Over 40 years later the arguments have hardly changed, although the jargon appears more sophisticated. In the late 1980s the justification for higher spending on the NHS made use of the 'efficiency-trap' argument; as the NHS became more efficient at its job – cutting unit costs and also increasing the number of patients it was able to treat – so total costs rose. In other words it was a victim of its own success.

More money, more patients

In terms of its success in attracting finance from the Treasury the record of the NHS since 1948 appears unparalleled. As Figure 3.1 shows, in cash terms, Exchequer expenditure on the Service has increased by nearly 6000 per cent – from £437 m. to over £26 000 m. in 1990–91. When some allowance is made for general inflation over the period the rise is more modest, but still stands at an impressive 330 per cent. This real rise in expenditure works out at an average annual increase of just under 4 per cent. However, this figure is based on a measure of inflation which inaccurately reflects the real inflationary pressures which face the NHS. The NHS 'buys' a unique 'basket of goods' – doctors, nurses, syringes, hospital beds,

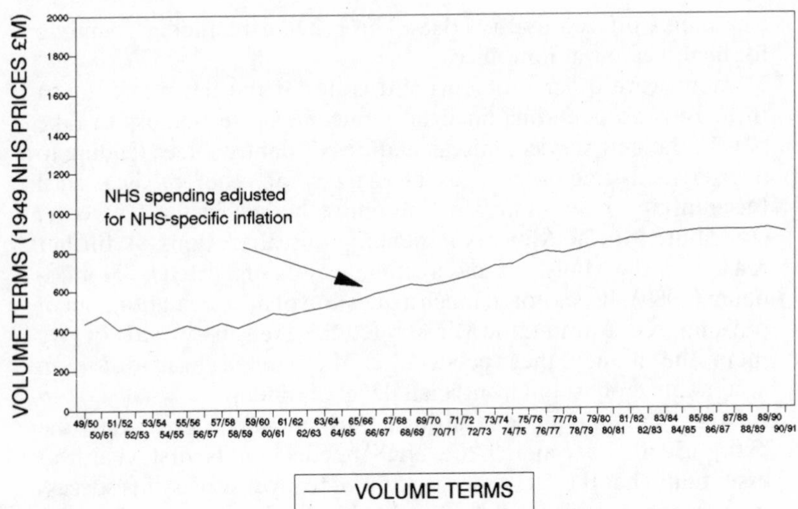

Figure 3.2 Total UK NHS expenditure: real spending (NHS pay and prices).

etc. It is the change in price of these inputs which is of relevance to the NHS. Taking into account health service-specific inflation reduces the NHS's real resource rise between 1949 and 1990 to around 115 per cent. This is equivalent to an average annual increase of about 1.9 per cent. But as Figure 3.2 makes clear, the change in real resources available to the NHS has not been as uniform as this average growth suggests.

The history of increased NHS spending is perhaps not as dramatic as it appeared at first sight. What the NHS did with the resources at its disposal is dramatic, however. Total discharges and deaths have increased from around 3 million in 1949–50 to about 8 million in 1989–90. Acute discharges and deaths per 1000 population nearly doubled and acute discharges and deaths per available bed increased 2.5 times. Similarly, new out-patient cases have doubled; the number of completed dental courses more than trebled; the number of dispensed prescriptions have also doubled and the total number of GPs has risen by nearly 50 per cent. It could be further argued that, not only has the NHS increased its *volume* of work, but also the *quality* of the services it delivers as new medical techniques were developed and medical knowledge improved.

So, in very broad terms, the NHS would appear to have done rather well financially through a combination of the improved efficiency with which it delivers its services plus increased real resources. The implication here that, because the NHS has done well that patients have also done well, is assumed for the time being. Whilst Illich's (1977) view of 'structural iatrogenesis' and 'maintenance medicine' (keeping workers minimally healthy for economic reasons) stretches conspiracy theory somewhat, the fact that health care exists in a *context*, that it is shaped and directed not only by some pure idea of medicine and healing but by a wide variety of forces is an important issue with repercussions for the way health care is delivered and financed. This is an important issue which is outwith the scope of this book, as is the assumption that, for example, the NHS can be congratulated for, amongst other things, doubling the number of prescriptions and increasing hospital throughput by 150 per cent since its inception. It should be borne in mind that more is not always good. However, to return to the main point: has there been any discernible pattern or trend in NHS financing since 1948?

Trends in the level of NHS spending

Identifying historical trends in the level of NHS financing can prove problematic depending on the data or statistic chosen. This was clear from the foregoing in which the tremendous rises in cash spending on the NHS start to look less momentous when account is taken of inflation. Not only that, but the smooth, almost exponential, growth in cash spending turns into a more erratic line when cash spending is deflated. And there are yet other ways of looking at total NHS spending – total spending per head of population, for example, or as a proportion of the UK's Gross National Product (GNP). The real or volume terms statistic can be extended to take account of what *ought* to have been spent if NHS expenditure was to have kept pace with changing health care demands, advances in medical technology, etc. This latter idea has formed the basis of most of the so-called 'underfunding calculations' carried out during the 1980s and is looked at more thoroughly in Chapter 4.

A perusal of the graphs detailing the various ways of measuring

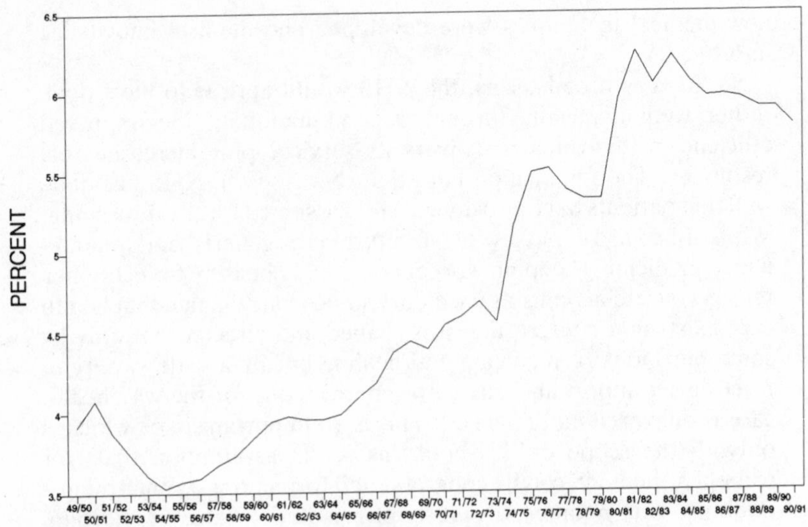

Figure 3.3 Total UK NHS expenditure as a percentage of GNP.
Source: OHE (1990).

the course of total NHS spending over the last 40 years reveals a number of points.

- Total cash spending on the NHS seems to divide into two periods – before 1970 and after 1970. In the former period, from 1948 to 1970, cash spending on the NHS remained fairly stable, rising from around £450 m. to just over £2000 m. (an increase of about 360 per cent). Between 1970 and 1990, however, expenditure rose from around £2000 m. to nearly £27 000 m. A rise of about 1250 per cent. It was in the early 1970s that cash spending began to rise almost exponentially for the next two decades.
- Making some allowance for inflation (using the general measure of Gross Domestic Product (GDP) at factor cost) produces a slightly different trend; still upward, but generally smoother, except for the last decade. Since 1949–50, spending appears to have trebled.
- As a percentage of GNP, NHS cash spending appears to have followed a much more erratic course. There is still a discernible upward trend, although by international comparisons, it is within a fairly narrow range (Figure 3.3).

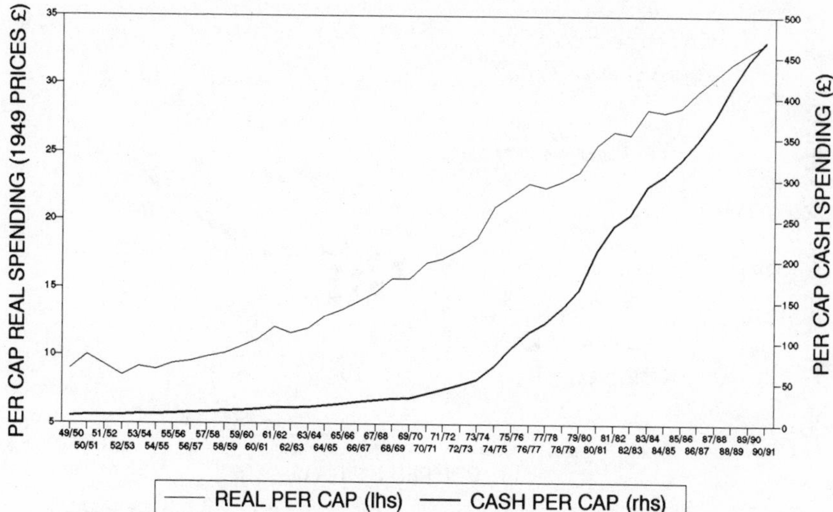

Figure 3.4 Total UK NHS expenditure: cash and real spending per head.
Source: OHE (1990).

- Cash and real spending per head show marked similarities with the graphs for total cash and real spending, although with a slight tendency to accentuate year on year changes (Figure 3.4).
- As can be seen from Figure 3.2, when the NHS-specific inflation rate is used to deflate total cash spending, spending since 1949–50 has doubled in real terms.

On their own, these graphs are perhaps of limited interest. They have their place in describing, from various viewpoints, what has happened in the past with NHS expenditure. Descriptive perhaps, but predictive? Although economists are fond of driving forward solely using the rear-view mirror (metaphorically speaking) it would be considered reckless, let alone careless, to predict future spending into the next decade simply by linearly extending the graphs forward another ten years. Such a crude extrapolation for total cash spending based on pre-1970 expenditure levels implies spending of £3000 m. in 1980 – whereas actual spending was £12 000 m. A greater sophistication is needed.

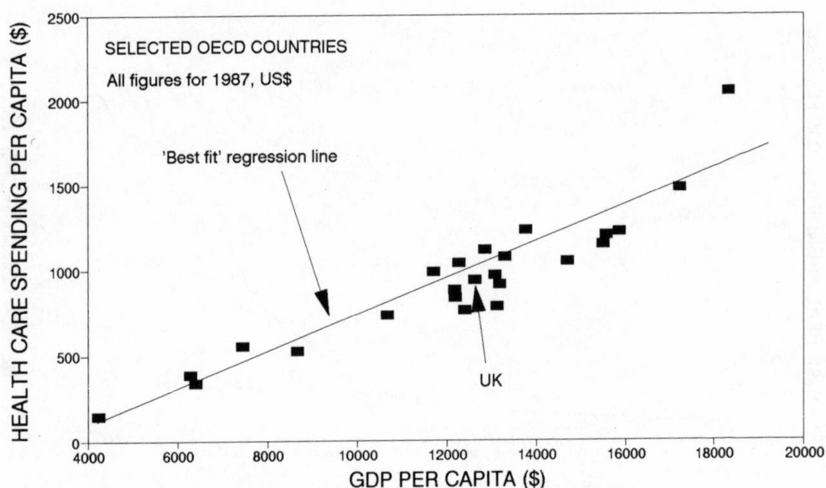

Figure 3.5 Relationship between wealth and health spending: international comparisons. All figures for 1987, in US$.

Source: Computed from OECD *Health Data File* (1989).

Economic models of an economic muddle?

Attempting to understand how and why health-care expenditures change over time, and in particular variations in spending between countries, has led to many different constructions of models of the behaviour of health-care expenditure. These models have tended to use cross-sectional international data and a handful of (hopefully) explanatory variables. All the models tend to suffer from one statistical problem or another, which can make interpretation of their results difficult. Nonetheless, certain patterns do emerge which shed some light on the historical trends in NHS spending over the last 40 years.

National income, as measured by GDP, for example, has been shown to correlate positively with health-care expenditure by all models, as is graphically shown by Figure 3.5. Not only that, but the actual numerical relationship appears to be remarkably stable or robust between models. Work by Gerdtham *et al.* (1988) confirms other work in this area and shows that every 1 per cent rise in GDP is associated with a 1.5 per cent rise in total health-care expenditure. Other studies (e.g. Leu, 1986) suggest perhaps that this income elasticity of 1.5 is on the high side. However, income elasticities

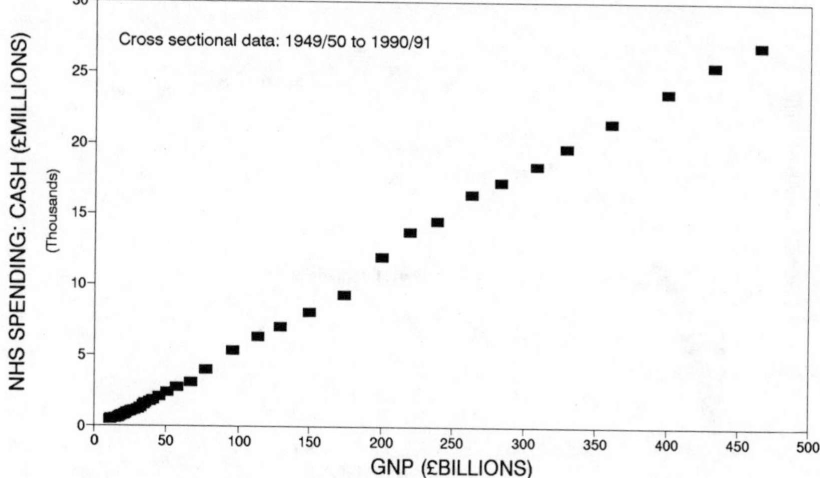

Figure 3.6 Relationship between NHS spending and UK Gross National Product.

seem to vary between 1 and 1.5. Rich countries spend more on health care as a proportion of their total income and per head of their populations. This does not mean that richer countries necessarily enjoy 'better' health-care systems (or, for that matter, better health). Higher spending on health care is not synonymous with higher levels of health or more efficient systems for delivering health care. Wealth does not always positively correlate with wisdom whereas it does seem to correlate with higher costs of health care provision (Parkin, 1989).

Parochially, the relationship between the UK's GNP (another way of measuring national income) and NHS spending over time appears very strong, as Figure 3.6 reveals. But more than this, there appears to be a positive relationship (although more erratic) between the proportion of the UK's wealth (as measured by GNP) and spending on the NHS, as illustrated by Figure 3.7. Although such relationships should be treated with care – spurious associations between variables can arise because of time trends – there are strong *a priori* reasons for believing in the positive link between wealth and health care spending. Exactly why richer countries spend more than poorer countries on health care, and why countries as they become richer should spend more is not actually explained by this income/health-care expenditure association. More is spent

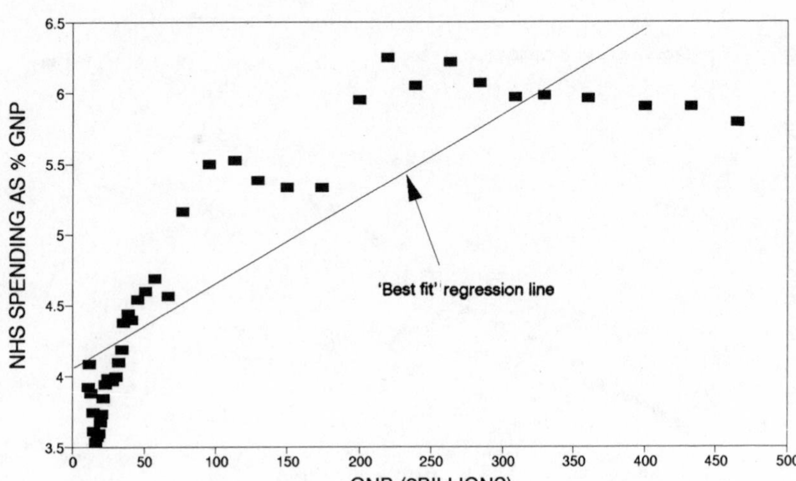

Figure 3.7 Relationship between NHS spending as a percentage of GNP and UK Gross National Product.

because more is available to be spent is only part of the explanation. There are other factors at work, some of which have been included in the models referred to above and others which would seem, *a priori*, to exert some influence but which have not been investigated as thoroughly.

International comparisons suggest that the type of health-care system, and particularly the type of financing methods these systems employ, are important in understanding variations in health-care spending. Leu (1986), for instance, differentiates between countries with a strong central control over health-care spending, those with more diffuse or more devolved control and 'direct democracies'. Unfortunately, elementary statistical problems arise; only two countries fit into Leu's first classification – New Zealand and the UK – and the direct democracy category boils down to a unique variable for Switzerland alone. Nevertheless, Leu produced some significant evidence to show that centralized control of health-care budgets (as in the UK) has a restrictive effect on total spending. He found that the presence of centralized control was associated with a 21 per cent fall in total spending. For direct democracies (i.e. Switzerland) the reduction was around 30 per cent.

Other influential factors which have been shown to be associated with health-care spending include: the proportion of the population under 15 years old; the proportion of the population living in cities of over 100 000 people; the share of public finance in total health-care spending and the share of public provision of health care in total provision. However, there has been conflicting evidence on the degree and even direction of influence of these factors.

It should be noted that these health-care expenditure models tend to look at total health-care spending, i.e. both public and private. Hence the inclusion in Leu's model of variables such as the proportion of public finance and public provision in total health-care spending and provision. These two variables are not relevant when just looking at NHS spending. However, they do become relevant when private health-care expenditure is included, as it is later in this chapter. One other issue which needs to be mentioned is the fact that these models use cross-sectional data (i.e. data for one year taken from many different countries) whereas here we are looking at time series data (i.e. data for many years taken from one country – the UK). Although these two data sets do not necessarily add up to the same results when modelled, and although particular (and different) statistical problems can arise with the two data sets, most of the results from the cross-sectional models (e.g. the influence of GDP and the type of health-care financing system, to choose the two most consistently significant variables) are also relevant to the time series data on the NHS.

Other models have specifically used time series data, combining knowledge about previous spending patterns with predictions of future changes in factors known to be associated with these spending patterns in order that they can produce estimates of future spending patterns. Propper and Upward (1990) explored models designed to predict the changes that might be expected to arise from alterations in the age structure of the population. Compared with known spending levels, their models' predictions produce under-estimates of NHS spending ranging from 7 to 23 per cent. With this qualification in mind, their models predict that demographic factors will tend to boost real NHS spending by between 1.4 and 5.3 per cent between 1991 and 2001. Other models (e.g. Bosanquet and Gray, 1989) have used more complicated designs than Propper and Upward, although results tend to be similar. Over the next ten years, changes in demography suggest that more will be spent on the NHS but at a decreasing rate.

Two other factors which have not been subjected to so much statistical scrutiny are the monopsony power of health-care systems (i.e. the power of large single buyers to influence the price they pay for their inputs or raw materials obtained from other suppliers) and Politics (with a capital P). Both these factors are particularly pertinent to the UK's record on NHS spending over the last 40 years.

The power of politics

By 'Politics' is meant the type of political party in power. This is not the same as the 'centralized control of health-care budgets' variable that Leu and others have included in their models (which were designed to differentiate between different forms of health-care system). Rather, it is a recognition of the fact that health-care systems with a centralized financial control (the NHS) are subject to wider macroeconomic (and social) policies of governments. This is not to suggest that NHS spending decisions are made only with reference to issues and policies totally unconnected with the NHS. Of course, these decisions are informed by, for example, predictive spending models such as Bosanquet and Gray's. However, actual NHS expenditures are not simply generated by algorithmic models, they are the outcome of a complex of political forces, which subsume such models.

Although cross-sectional expenditure models have shown that centralized control tends to contain rises in spending – and hence it can be said that without such a system in the UK over the last 40 years, health-care spending would have been higher now than it actually is – such a prediction could not have been made using time series data for NHS spending over the last 40 years because the centralized control variable itself has not changed. However, governments and government economic policy has. By including some variable representing 'Politics' (e.g. the type of political party in power, for example) the political influence over NHS spending over the last 40 years may be captured in a way Leu's and others' models (which use international cross-sectional data) cannot.

In simple terms, all that is being suggested is that it is more than likely that the history of NHS spending is linked to the history of political control in the UK since 1948.

Wells' (1991) dissection of NHS expenditure into the seven political administrations which have, at various times since the

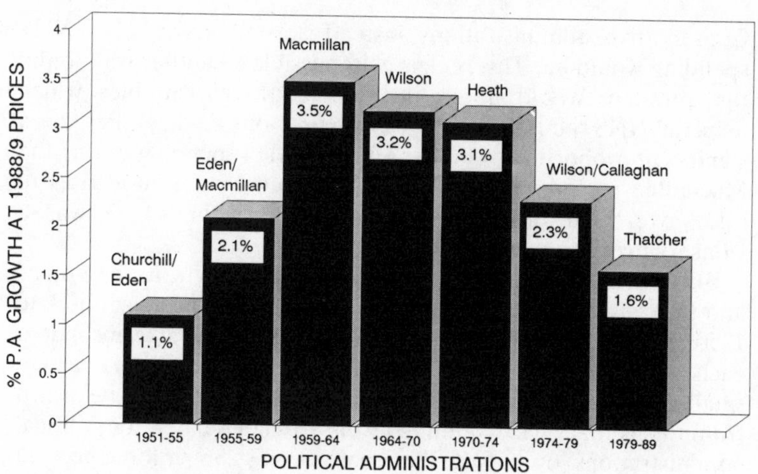

Figure 3.8 Total NHS spending: percentage real growth per annum.
Source: Wells (1991).

beginning of the 1950s, controlled NHS spending has revealed a pattern, but between *administrations* and not *parties* in power. Figure 3.8 shows that the average annual change in total real NHS spending (i.e. adjusted for NHS pay and price inflation) varied from 1.1 per cent in the Churchill/Eden period of the first half of the 1950s, to 3.5 per cent over the first half of the 1960s during Macmillan's administration. So, during the period of office of two Conservative administrations, the growth in spending on the NHS was the highest and the lowest. Statistically, seven observations is a rather low number from which to draw any robust conclusions. Even if it had turned out to be the case that during the two terms of Labour administration, NHS spending had been at its highest, the difference in the average annual increases between Labour and Conservative periods of office would have needed to be exceptionally large in order to guarantee a reasonably significant statistical association between spending and type of party in power. The lack of observations works the other way, of course. Because there appears to be no clear association between the type of party in power and NHS spending does not mean that such an association does not exist. One way of resolving this equivocation would be to re-run, say, the Wilson and Wilson/Callaghan periods of office with

Conservative administrations instead and then see what NHS spending would be. This is clearly impossible. Another way round this problem would be to include additional variables which 'explain' NHS spending levels (as with previous models). Perhaps a significant proportion of the large rise in NHS spending during the Macmillan period would then be explained by the large rises in GDP over that time, rather than the fact that there was a Conservative administration in power.

But there is a more noticeable trend apparent from the graph, and that is the decreasing growth in NHS spending since the late 1950s/early 1960s. NHS spending still increased in real terms, but in each successive period of political administration the rise was smaller. Statistical qualifications aside, one conclusion to be drawn from this is that NHS spending levels are independent of political administrations, or at least, there have been stronger influences on spending levels. This is not, however, a very robust conclusion, and would appear at odds with the fact that political administrations do have direct control over NHS spending.

One buyer, one price

As Culyer (1990) has noted, the degree of influence of monopsony power over health-care expenditure has not been well studied. This seems strange given that there is a strong *a priori* case for arguing that the monopsony power of, say, the NHS (particularly over pay, which constitutes over a half of total NHS spending and 16–17 per cent of all central government spending) has tended to contain rises in spending. In a qualitative analysis of the 1990 NHS Act's partial deregulation of the health-care labour market, Mayston (1990) has concluded that a more competitive labour market (i.e. a reduction in the NHS's monopsony power) would lead to a rise in wage costs. In short, the NHS benefits financially from its monopsonistic position. For the ancillary staff working for one-third of the national average male wage, the fact that their foregone pay has enabled the NHS to employ more staff, buy more equipment and keep down costs is perhaps not so obvious an advantage.

Two services, not one

Finally, it is worth noting a trend which tends to get buried or at least obscured by concentration on the NHS as a whole and not as

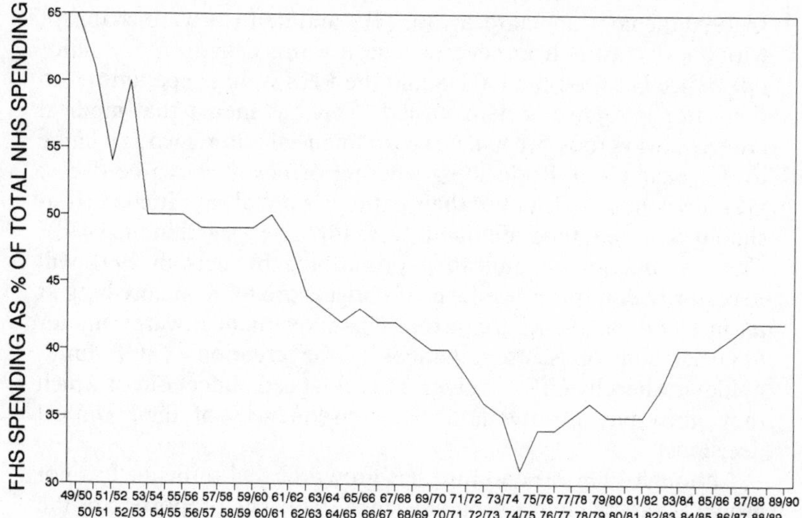

Figure 3.9 Ratio of family health service to hospital and community health service spending.
Source: OHE (1990).

the dichotomy between the hospital and community health services (HCHS) on the one hand, and family health services (FHS) on the other. Since 1949, there has been a trend away from expenditure on the FHS and towards spending on the HCHS which has only latterly been reversed, as Figure 3.9 shows. In 1949, total expenditure on the FHS was around one-third of total spending on the NHS (the ratio of HCHS to FHS spending was 65 per cent). By 1990, this proportion had fallen to a quarter (a ratio of 42 per cent). It was only in the mid-1970s, with the slow down in spending on the HCHS that the FHS started to catch up as a proportion of total spending.

The FHS are provided by doctors – general practitioners (GPs) – dentists and other health-care professionals, all of whom are independent contractors, not employees of the NHS. The services they provide are paid for by central government (not local District Health Authorities) using a variety of payment methods – fee per item of service and capitation. This means that GPs' incomes are derived partly from a standard payment for the number of people on their lists and partly from work they carry out for those people.

In 1990 the contractual terms for GPs and dentists were changed, with a move away from fee per item towards capitation. A major difference between the HCHS and the FHS is that expenditure on the latter is relatively demand-led. This has meant that medical criteria always took precedence over financial criteria when it came to, for example, GPs deciding whether or not to prescribe drugs; GPs' demands on behalf of their patients were always funded (if, it should be noted, those demands were for services within the FHS). The introduction of indicative prescribing budgets in 1991 will necessarily dull this precedence if budgets are to mean anything at all in terms of financial control. This movement towards tighter financial control is strengthened by the creation of GP fund-holders, whereby GPs are given a tax-financed budget out of which they must pay for the financial consequences of their clinical decisions.

Although FHS expenditure has grown in real terms, it has not grown as fast as HCHS spending since 1949. The proportion of the total NHS budget which has been controlled centrally (i.e. not so overtly driven by demand) has grown over the last 40 years.

Trends in the source of NHS spending

Although the NHS has been and remains overwhelmingly funded from one source – general taxation – there have been some noticeable changes over the last 40 years. In the first few years of the NHS's existence, 100 per cent of its finance was provided by general taxation. From the early 1950s, however, other sources of finance were introduced. NHS contributions, local authority rates and direct patient charges made up nearly 18 per cent of total NHS spending in 1951, for example. By 1963 these sources had grown to nearly 33 per cent of total spending. With the transfer of health services funded and run by local authorities to NHS funding and control in 1974, the proportion of total spending financed from general taxation stood at over 90 per cent. Since then, however, tax funding has fallen to around 77 per cent with the remaining 23 per cent coming from NHS contributions, patient charges and various forms of income generation. Table 3.1 shows the sources of finance for the NHS between 1949 and 1988. Table 3.2 gives a more recent and more detailed breakdown of financing sources (including receipts from asset sales, for example), for the years 1978–79 and 1990–91. So, although general taxation has been and remains the

Table 3.1 UK NHS: Sources of finance

Year	*Taxation (%)*	*NHS contributions (%)*	*Local Health Authority* (%)*	*Patient payments (%)*
1949	100.0	–	–	–
1950	100.0	–	–	–
1951	82.3	8.3	8.2	1.2
1952	80.2	8.0	8.4	3.4
1953	79.9	7.5	8.2	4.4
1954	80.0	7.3	8.3	4.4
1955	80.4	6.9	8.4	4.3
1956	81.2	6.2	8.4	4.2
1957	79.4	7.6	8.3	4.6
1958	74.2	13.0	8.5	4.3
1959	73.6	13.7	8.6	4.1
1960	74.4	13.1	8.5	4.0
1961	72.0	14.5	8.9	4.7
1962	70.0	15.9	9.3	4.8
1963	70.7	15.1	9.5	4.7
1964	71.8	14.2	9.5	4.5
1965	75.1	12.1	9.7	2.5
1966	77.0	11.6	9.4	2.1
1967	77.6	10.5	9.8	2.1
1968	76.6	10.4	9.8	3.2
1969	78.8	10.4	7.3	3.6
1970	79.9	10.2	6.6	3.3
1971	80.2	10.0	6.6	3.2
1972	81.3	8.8	6.6	3.3
1973	82.3	7.9	6.7	3.2
1974	91.0	5.9	–	2.6
1975	89.4	8.5	–	2.0
1976	88.4	9.5	–	2.0
1977	88.2	9.6	–	2.2
1978	88.4	9.5	–	2.1
1979	88.3	9.5	–	2.2
1980	88.9	8.7	–	2.5
1981	87.7	9.8	–	2.8
1982	86.2	11.0	–	2.8
1983	86.5	10.7	–	2.8
1984	86.5	10.8	–	2.7
1985	86.1	11.0	–	2.8
1986	85.8	11.4	–	2.8
1987	84.5	12.7	–	2.7
1988	82.6	14.6	–	2.8

Source: OHE (1990)

* *Note:* Local Health Authorities existed to 1974. From 1974, services were transferred to the NHS.

Table 3.2 NHS sources of finance: percentages of total year for the UK

Fund	*Consolidated contributions*	*NHS*	*Charges*	*Miscellaneous*
1978–79	88.0	9.6	2.1	0.3
1979–80	87.9	9.6	2.2	0.3
1980–81	89.1	8.2	2.4	0.3
1981–82	87.8	9.4	2.5	0.3
1982–83	85.7	11.3	2.7	0.3
1983–84	85.8	11.0	2.8	0.4
1984–85	85.6	11.1	2.8	0.5
1985–86	85.6	11.0	2.7	0.7
1986–87	84.4	11.7	2.9	1.0
1987–88	83.0	13.0	2.8	1.2
1988–89*	80.9	14.5	2.9	1.7
1989–90*	78.3	16.2	4.0	1.5
1990–91*	77.0	15.0	6.5	1.5

Source: 1978–79 to 1989–90, House of Commons (1990); 1990–91, DoH (1991)

* *Note:* Figures for 1988 to 1991 are estimates.

main source of funding for the health services in the UK, it has by no means remained constant. Moreover, there have been considerable changes in the last decade. For example, whilst the 300–400 per cent real rise in prescription charges since 1952 has been considerably offset by the rise in exemptions from charges (now standing at about 85 per cent of all prescriptions cashed), the privatization of sight tests (except for some groups such as children, those with low incomes, etc.) has shifted a portion of previously tax-funded expenditure onto individuals. The response of the public to this has been disputed, but a not unnatural outcome has been a drop in the number of sight tests (a rational economic reaction to an increase in price).

Asset sales

Another source of (finite) income for the NHS which has come to prominence in the last few years has been money raised from selling surplus land and buildings. In 1990, land and estate sales constituted 20 per cent of the English HCHS's capital allocation; in 1980 it was 3

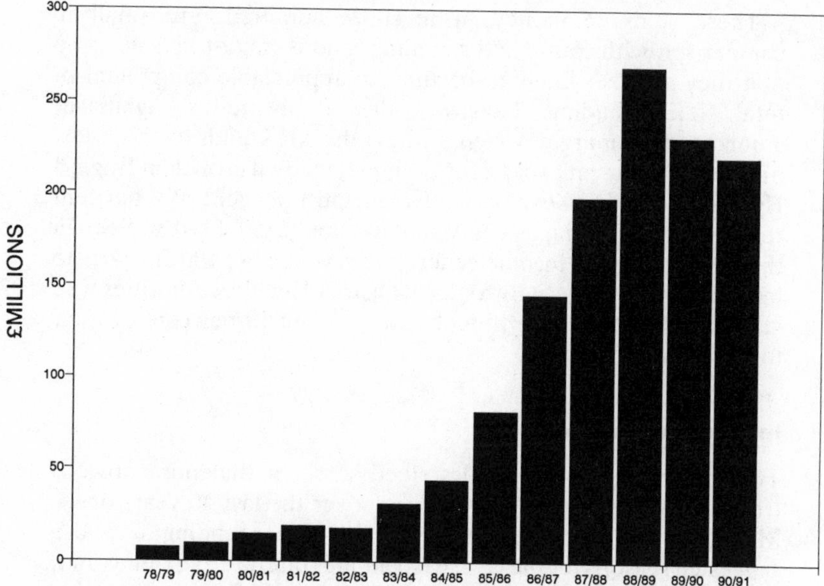

Figure 3.10 Receipts from sale of land and buildings, England.
Sources: House of Commons (1990), DoH (1991).

per cent. Figure 3.10 shows that income from the sale of land and buildings has increased by nearly 31 times between 1978–79 and 1989–90. As Mark Twain stated, 'they ain't making land no more'. Implicit in this observation are two truisms: first, the tendency for land prices to rise in the long run, and secondly the inevitability of limited supplies reaching their limit. There are clearly limits to the amount of revenue the NHS can generate from sales of land and property.

Income generation

Whilst the NHS has been busily divesting itself of a finite resource, it has also been busy generating income from renewable sources. New income generation schemes currently produce around £60–70 m. a year for the NHS. Cumulatively, income from flower shops, cafeterias in hospitals and the like amounts to nearly £100 m., and it is growing.

These sums of money, it must be admitted, are small in comparison with total NHS spending, and it cannot be suggested that they are ever likely to become an appreciable component of total NHS spending. However, they do represent significant amounts at the margin, which is where the NHS tends to exist most of the time. In recent years, for example, the real growth in English HCHS funding has been between zero and 1 per cent. A 1 per cent real growth in funding is equivalent to about £150–£170 m. Seen in this light, recurring income generation revenue of £100 m. starts to look important, especially for local District Health Authorities who are able to generate anything between 5 and 10 per cent of their total allocation.

Interpreting the trends

The foregoing has briefly described some of the more obvious trends in NHS funding and financing over the last 40 years or so. Modelling the determinants of health-care spending has also suggested reasons for the level of spending. Interpreting trends and, more importantly, deciding on the extent to which they determine the future is difficult. One of the main reasons for this difficulty is that the NHS stands at a turning point created by the reforms of various White Papers published between 1988 and 1990. These reforms, as Chapter 2 noted, contain the seeds of some great changes in the structure and economic environment of the NHS which mark a break with the past. However, this does not necessarily mean that there is no continuity with the past trends outlined above, or that some useful predictive analysis cannot be done (such as Mayston's on the deregulation of the health-care labour market).

More money to spend means more money to spend?

Leaving aside the problem of recent policy changes regarding the NHS, there are a number of points which emerge from the pattern of historical spending on the Service. First, national income or per capita GNP appears to be one of the most important indicators of the total level of spending. If per capita GNP increases over the next decade then there is a significant likelihood that a corresponding rise in NHS spending will also be apparent. Secondly, however, centralized control of health-care spending means that any growth in total expenditure is likely to be undramatic. Thirdly, demographic change, and in particular changes in the number and proportion in the total population of elderly people, will tend to add considerable pressure to demands for increased spending levels. Whilst the growth in the total numbers and proportion of the group who use health-care services in greatest disproportion to their numbers (and tax-generating capacity) – the elderly – will require an increase in real resources, the rate of increase will slow over the next decade. There are, of course, other trends which may well turn out to be significant. For example, the combined demand pressures of demography, medical advance and changing patterns of disease may add weight to the small trends in diversification of sources of funding for the NHS as governments attempt to decentralize the increasingly intractable health-care funding problem by spreading the responsibility for funding more widely.

Looking at the past quite obviously gives an imperfect view of the future. Better understanding of the reasons for historical trends in NHS spending and financing, means that predictions for the future are switched from extrapolations of the direct financial trends to extrapolations of associated or perhaps causal factors, such as GNP or the population of elderly people. These 'explanatory' factors can be predicted with varying degrees of accuracy. To a large extent, however, predictions tend to be qualitative rather than quantitative. Examination of past trends tend to give indications of possible changes in the direction of future spending (i.e. up or down) rather than accurate predictions of the actual size of changes. This is particularly true for relatively recent trends or policy changes. Mayston's analysis of a possible rise in wage inflation (and hence total expenditure, but not real expenditure) following abandonment of centralized wage bargaining in the NHS is an example of the latter.

There is another problem, however, and this is the apparent determinism of the trends/modelling approach to prediction. The connection between, say, GNP and NHS spending is not inevitable; we do not *have* to spend more if GNP per capita rises and we do not *have* to spend less if it falls. Ultimately, what the trends and models reveal is some of the information needed in order to make a decision about the future. The rest of this information (indeed the great bulk of it) will come, as Culyer (1990) and many others have pointed out, from detailed cost-benefit analysis at the macro level in terms of resource commitment choices between public and private expenditure, between defence, education, housing and health-care spending, etc. And at the micro level, funding priorities will be characterized by choices between different health-care services and treatments.

THE RISE AND RISE OF THE PRIVATE SECTOR

Whilst it is evident that health care in the UK has been dominated by public provision and public finance, it is equally clear that individual or private provision and finance has made a significant contribution to what may be termed 'the global health-care sector'. There are some problems in defining what constitutes private health care: should my purchase of a packet of cough sweets count as 'private health-care' expenditure? (maybe it should be counted as negative expenditure given the probable effect of the sweets on my dental state); should the time I spend swimming somehow be valued and counted? More seriously, where does the unpaid (but enormously costly) work of carers (relatives, friends, neighbours, etc.) fit in? In fact, an argument exists for counting everything human beings do, buy and work for which is not explicitly the NHS as contributing in some way to private health care. Defining the private health-care sector as 'not the NHS' is, however, not particularly helpful (or manageable). A more conventional set of boundaries to the private health-care sector is used by Laing (1989). He includes more recognizably health-care-related sectors such as acute care, long-term care of the elderly, physically handicapped, pharmaceuticals and so on. Data limitations notwithstanding, it is these areas which will be examined here.

Obtaining long-term trends on private health-care spending and financing is not as straightforward as for public spending (although changes in definitions in national accounts make the latter difficult enough to compile). Virtually all the figures quoted here have been taken from Laing (1989, 1990), the Office of Health Economics (1990) and other *ad hoc* sources to try and build up as full a historic picture as possible.

Trends in the level of spending

Between 1972 and 1989, spending on private acute care rose by 2800 per cent in cash terms, or 442 per cent in real terms after allowing for inflation as measured by the retail prices index (Laing, 1990)

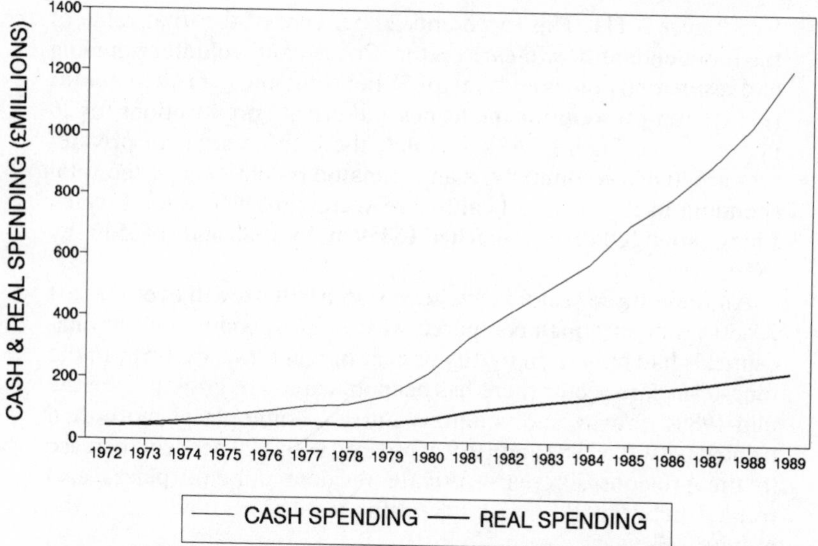

Figure 3.11 Total UK private acute care expenditure: cash and real spending (1972 prices).

Source: Laing (1990).

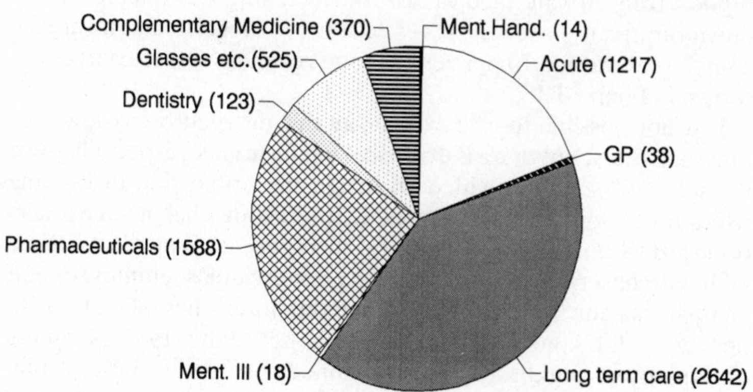

Figure 3.12 Private health care: spending breakdown by sector (total = £6535 m.).

Source: Laing (1990).

(see Figure 3.11). This represents 20 per cent of the total value of the independent health-care sector. Private and voluntary nursing and residential homes account for 38 per cent, and over-the-counter (OTC) non-prescription medicines and private prescriptions for 26 per cent (see Figure 3.12). In total, these three areas of private-sector activity accounted for an estimated 84 per cent of the total spending in the private health-care sector in 1988, a total which Laing estimated to have reached £5459 m. by 1988 and £6535 m. by 1989.

All these three sectors have seen significant growth over the last 20–30 years, although compared with 1973, spending on pharmaceuticals had only risen by 10 per cent in real terms by 1988. In the long-term care sector there has been an explosive growth since the mid-1980s: private and voluntary nursing-home places more than trebled between 1984 and 1989 compared with a 20 per cent increase in the previous six years; private residential home places also trebled between 1984 and 1989, after a similarly low rise in the previous six years.

Sources of funding

The sources of finance for the various sectors which make up the private health-care sector differ. The acute sector (providing specialized, non-emergency, mostly surgical, care) is principally funded from private medical insurance. Laing's estimated breakdown of private hospitals' revenue sources suggests that insurance contributes around 70 per cent of total revenue. Other sources are shown in Figure 3.13.

It is not possible to calculate easily this detailed breakdown for previous years, but there is evidence that insurance, especially since the late 1970s, has provided an increasing proportion of funding while other sources have declined. Interesting changes have also occurred within the private medical-insurance market. Of the three main purchasers of medical insurance – individuals, employees and companies – the number of individual purchasers has fallen from 43 per cent of total purchasers in 1972 to 27 per cent in 1987. Numbers of employee purchasers has remained relatively static, while company purchasers have increased from 40 to 56 per cent (Propper and Maynard, 1989). Laing points out, however, that data from the 1986 *General Household Survey* (*GHS*) suggests that about 20 per cent of company purchasers are in fact employees who pay the full

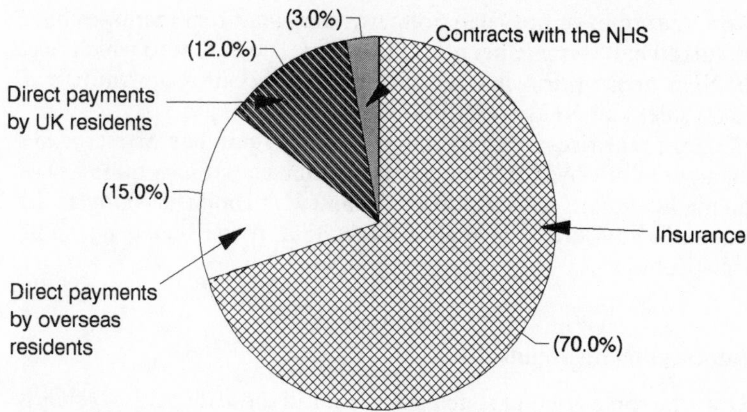

Figure 3.13 Private health care: sources of funding.
Source: Laing (1990).

premiums themselves – their employers merely providing an administrative 'umbrella' for the purchase.

When it comes to private nursing, residential and long-stay hospital care for the elderly, chronically sick and disabled, insurance has traditionally been a negligible or non-existent source of funding. In 1988, over 40 per cent of this sector's revenue was funded from the public purse (i.e. taxation) via the Department of Social Security (DSS) in the form of income support. The remaining 60 per cent came from direct payments by the users of private long-term care services. The tremendous growth in this sector from the late 1970s onwards was the result of a combination of factors: an increase in demand (more elderly people); static or falling public supply and vastly increased public funding for the private sector via income support from the DSS. As Bosanquet and Gray (1989) have pointed out, nobody, at the beginning of the 1980s, would have predicted (or perhaps desired?) the effect that public subsidies of private health care would have on provision. Given hindsight, it may have been preferable to spend the £1 bn. currently channelled to the private long-term care sector in another direction.

Pharmaceutical expenditure is largely made up from OTC sales (84 per cent in 1988). The remainder is accounted for by private prescriptions. The historical trends in private pharmaceutical expenditure have not been dramatic, and what real increases have occurred have largely been in OTC sales. The extent to which rises in NHS prescription charges have brought about a substitution in OTC sales and NHS prescriptions is difficult to estimate.

Large real rises in charges have made a number of medicines cheaper to buy over the counter rather than via prescription. As not all medicines are 'prescription only' and with chemists acting as the patient's adviser, it is highly likely that there has been some substitution.

Interpreting the trends

Drawing some general conclusions from all these disparate trends is not easy. There seem to be a whole variety of factors at work influencing the historic spending and financing patterns in private health care. However, Laing has suggested that there are four main factors which, in concert and opposition, can be shown to have exerted most influence:

- The limits the NHS sets to its responsibilities: the NHS does not meet all demands. Either deliberately selecting certain forms of treatments and excluding others, or by default (lack of funding).
- The lack of a traditional involvement in certain modes of health care: for example, the NHS does not provide nursing homes on the private sector model.
- The limits of medical-insurance cover: for example, maternity is not covered and other restrictions exist (based on age, condition, etc).
- The marginal cost of care outside the NHS: where lower marginal costs of choosing private over public care exist, the private sector flourishes.

But to these can be added other significant factors. How the NHS is perceived, particularly the quality of service and waiting lists (too often numbers of patients waiting rather than the more relevant factor of length of time the individual has to wait) have been shown to be significant issues taken into consideration by people who choose to 'go private' (Higgins, 1988). Private medical insurance is a primary source of finance for the private health-care sector, but it is not just the limits of cover offered which affects the demand for insurance (and hence, indirectly, the demand for private care, although the two are not perfectly synonymous). Propper and Maynard (1989) have shown that medical insurance is 'price inelastic'. That is, a 10 per cent change in its price tends to bring about a change in quantity demanded of less than 10 per cent. This suggests that the purchasers of medical insurance are relatively insensitive to price changes. And the possible consequences of this are that providers of private health care could raise their prices and insurance companies could pass on the higher costs in the form of higher premiums with comparative impunity in terms of loss of demand. Expenditure in the private sector rises, but as a result of increased costs, not additional demand. Finally, the role of government cannot be overlooked. Policy changes regarding NHS funding, taxation, and attitudes and actions on the social, economic and legal fronts all exert influence over the financing of, and expenditure on, private health care.

CONCLUSION

This chapter has compressed much statistical information into a short space and it has not been possible (or in fact the intention) to look at all the many issues raised by an examination of historical patterns in health-care spending in the UK. The main purpose was to see what could be learned from looking at the past which might help inform a view about what will happen in the future.

It should be clear that the historical pattern of financing – both in terms of levels of funding and its sources – have arisen for a variety of reasons, from deliberate and accidental policy decisions by government through to underlying trends in demography which inform individual and collective decisions about health-care financing. Where the historical perspective is most useful is the data it provides to construct models which go some way to 'explaining' past trends, and which then, by a leap of inductive faith, go some way to predicting what perhaps is most likely to happen in the future. The statistical models described in this chapter are, however, not very robust if used for this purpose. Their main aim (apart from pure description) is to suggest what the future *could* be *if* certain things happen (an increase in the number of elderly or a fall in national income, say, is likely to lead to a certain level of health-care funding).

The specification of these models is not perfect however, and statistical methods have their limitations when it comes to coping with rare events such as the dramatic reforms of the NHS currently underway. What these quantitative models need is a hefty injection of qualitative data or information: an interpretation of more recent policy changes and financial trends.

4

THE RIGHT LEVEL OF FUNDING

If there is one statistic with which the health of the NHS is (at least popularly) judged, it is the level of funding it receives. Anecdotal and survey evidence of financial difficulties in the NHS grab the headlines, polarize the arguments and cloud the issues. For those in charge of the public purse, defence of past spending records comes first, followed by some blame shifting to NHS management for poor financial control. For others it is underfunding which is to blame. The underlying arguments of the former are based on cost minimization, whilst those of the latter are based on benefit maximization. Neither are solidly based, however: the cost minimizers presumably only being happy when the logical conclusion of their argument has been reached and costs equal zero, and the benefit maximizers only ceasing to voice their concerns about underfunding when all the nation's productive capacity is devoted to health care.

These straw men may get blown away in the wind, but the kernel of both beliefs tend to remain. Identifying the chaff is fairly easy; obviously we do not want to spend everything we have on the NHS – we want to devote some of our energies, resources, etc. to other things as well (food springs to mind). And whilst there may be some die-hard NHS cost minimizers, it would take a government hell bent on self-destruction to seriously heed the advice to go for maximum cost minimization. Given the existence of state funding of a health-care service (albeit a changing and evolving service) and given that the funding extremes (everything or nothing) are untenable positions, only two possibilities remain – one theoretical and almost certainly unattainable, the other pragmatic with virtually its sole defence being its attainability.

In theory, the right level of funding for the NHS is reached when to spend just one more pound on the service would produce benefits to society which would be just equivalent if that pound were spent on something else (education, say, or defence, or food). Stated in these broad terms (what exactly is meant by 'benefits'?) the theory is unassailable. The problem is that it is also impossible to put into practice. One stumbling block is the problem of measuring all alternative uses of every pound in a commensurate way. Money could be used of course, but how is the output of the NHS (healthiness?), or of education (intelligence?), or of defence (peace?) to be converted into pounds and pence? Another problem is knowing where the NHS is on the curve showing the marginal rate of return to health-care investment. Figure 4.1 shows this. Is it at point A (as those who argue the NHS is underfunded would assert), in which case more investment (higher spending) would produce a good return? Or is it at point B, the flat of the curve, where little is to be gained from more investment? Or is it at point C, where higher spending, pound for pound, will bring lower returns?

It may at first seem paradoxical, but the enormous difficulties of ascertaining where the NHS currently resides on this curve, calculating what the trade offs are between health and other forms of spending, should not be used as an excuse not to carry out work in this area, however. This is because there are benefits to be had even with some limited success in tackling these and other problems associated with this particular theoretical approach to the problem of the right level of funding for the NHS. This is perhaps the economist's interpretation of the notion that it is better to travel hopefully than to arrive! But meanwhile, back at the hospital, patients are waiting for their operations, surgeons, nurses, porters are waiting to be paid and the crumbling floor of the catering department is waiting to be resurfaced. The theory is fine, but the NHS and all who depend on it cannot afford to sit around paralysed, waiting for a practical, even just a partial, solution to the theory. Budgets need to be set. A pragmatic and practical solution needs to be found.

The words 'pragmatic' and 'practical' are more often than not used as euphemisms which conceal assumptions so broad, so extensive and so lacking in any real justification at all that one may wonder on the veracity of the actions they endorse or propose. However, as may have become clear above, the more perfect alternative to the pragmatic or practical solution to the question of

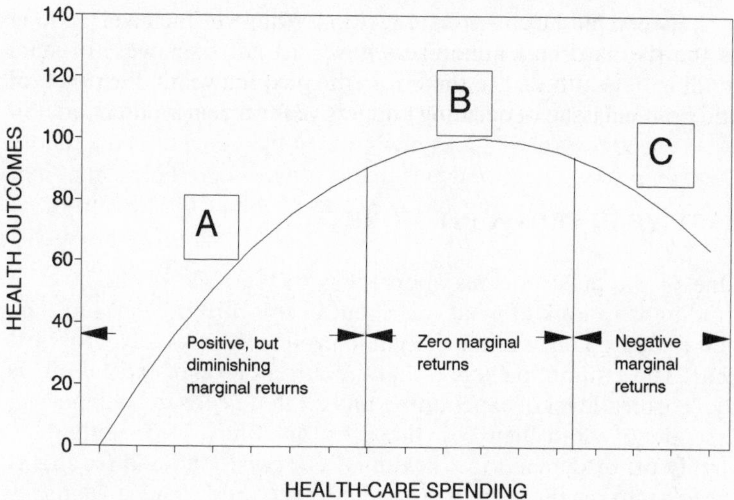

Figure 4.1 Diminishing returns on health-care spending.

Source: Culyer (1989).

the right level of funding for the NHS is currently unable to get off its theoretical starting blocks. In view of this, and, as has been said, the fact that life and the NHS must go on, the pragmatic solution should not be too quickly dismissed or despised for its potential lack of purity, as, for the time being at least, 'it's all we've got'.

This chapter will critically examine four practical approaches to the problem of determining the level of state funding for the NHS. (They are specific approaches to the problem of state funding of any health-care system.):

- Incremental funding
- Incremental funding linked to affordability
- International comparisons
- Democratic decision

For other forms of funding (private medical insurance, for example) the problem or question of the level of health-care funding becomes a private, microeconomic decision which is resolved by ability to pay. However, this is not to say that there is no interaction or trade off between public and private sectors. Whatever the level (so long as the die-hard cost minimizers have not got their way) of state funding of health care in the UK in the next ten years, the practical and political issue of deciding budgets year on year will remain.

LAST YEAR PLUS A BIT MORE

One of the most obvious approaches to the issue of the level of funding is to look at what was spent in the current year and then make some changes at the margin to produce a new budget for next year. The assumption here is that the current level of expenditure is the 'correct' level of expenditure and all that needs to be done is to first identify and then cost those factors which affect either the supply of, or demand for, health-care services and add (subtract) these to (from) the current year's budget to produce next year's.

This idea of isolating factors affecting health-care expenditure

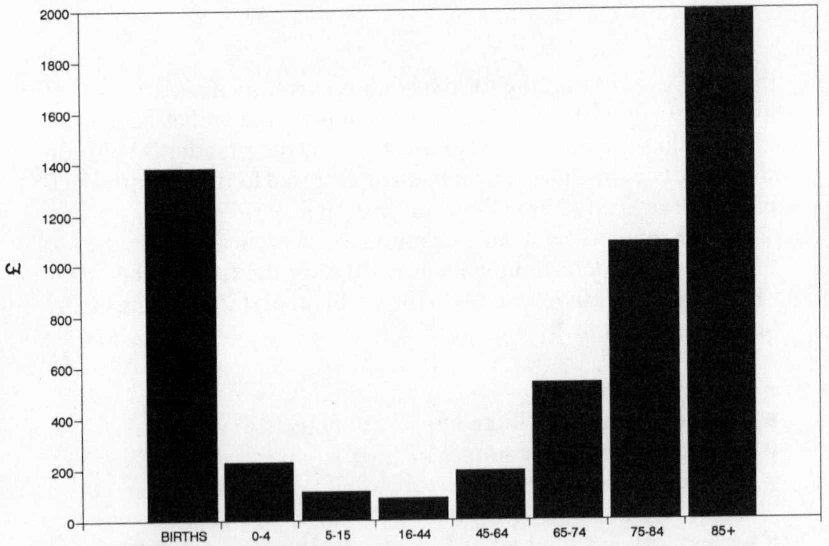

Figure 4.2 Gross current spending per head per age on hospital and community health service, England, 1988–89.

Source: DoH (1991).

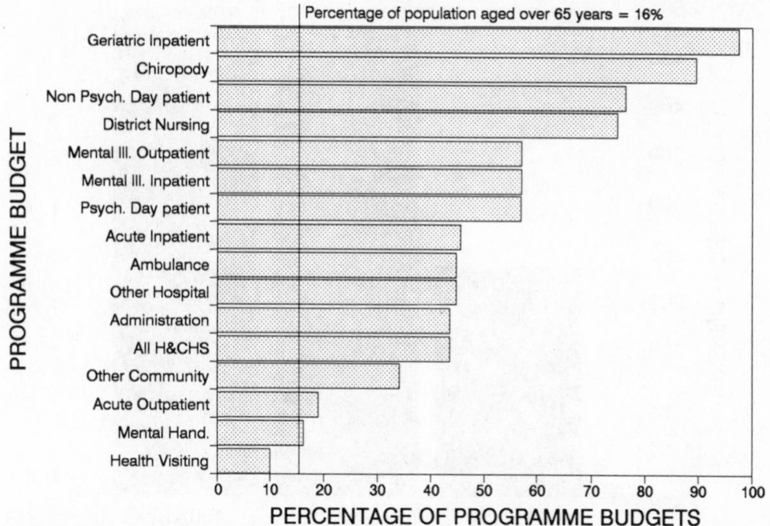

Figure 4.3 Percentage of hospital and community health service spending devoted to over-65-year-olds: England, HCHS, 1986–87.

Source: Bosanquet and Gray (1989).

recalls the descriptive spending models of Chapter 3. And indeed, some of the same factors crop up here in the prescriptive approaches to funding.

Funding demographic change

One particular factor which recurs in government statements of the objectives of the NHS is the need for the Service to meet the growing health care demands of the elderly. As an NHS user group, elderly people are very important. In financial terms NHS spending per head on people aged over 75 years is around 9–10 times greater than on people aged 16–64 years (Department of Health, 1991, and Figure 4.2). Splitting up the NHS by programme (i.e. acute care, geriatrics, mental handicap, etc.) and age group reveals that, for example, over 45 per cent of spending on acute in-patient care is devoted to people aged over 65 years, 58 per cent of mental illness spending, 75 per cent of district nursing expenditure and so on, as Figure 4.3 shows. In part this reflects the volume of NHS resource

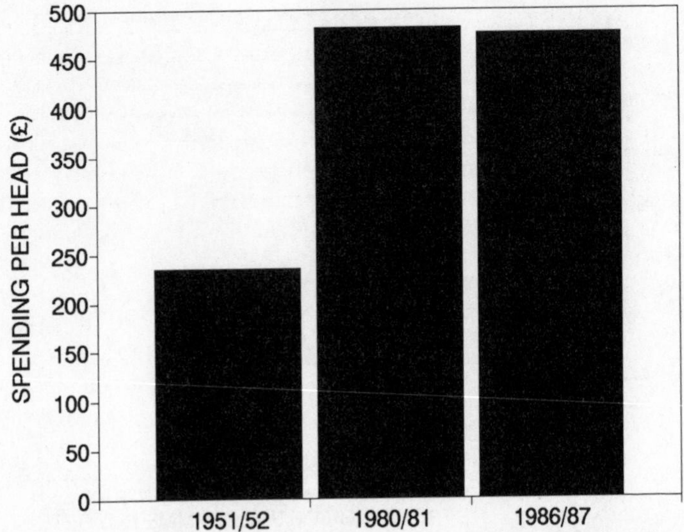

Figure 4.4 Estimated NHS expenditure per head for over-75-year-olds.
Source: Bosanquet and Gray (1989).

use by the elderly. But when allowance is made for the greater intensity of resource use arising from generally longer and more frequent lengths of stay, more complex interventions, etc, nearly 57 per cent of acute in-patient spending is devoted to people aged over 65 years. So, although as a group the elderly make up a comparatively small proportion of the total population (around 16 per cent), they make greater and more intensive use of the NHS than any other age group.

It is interesting to note that this has not always been the case. Estimates of the proportion of the NHS budget devoted to the over-65-year-olds (Abel-Smith and Titmuss, 1956; Bosanquet and Gray, 1989) show that expenditure attributable to this group has risen from 20 per cent in 1951–52 to nearly 50 per cent in 1988. And in per capita terms, spending on the over-75-year-olds has risen from around twice the average for all age groups to almost five times the average over the same period (see Figure 4.4). These changes reflect in part the higher priority accorded to the elderly, changes in the nature of health care, and, importantly, changes in the patterns of disease and demography over the last 30–40 years.

It is clear that responding to changes in demography, in particular changes in the population and proportion of the elderly and very elderly, is an important task for the NHS. This was identified by Abel-Smith and Titmuss in the early 1950s and was resurrected by health economists and others in the 1970s and 1980s, paralleling concerns about the growth in the number of the elderly – the 'greying of the population' – and contributing to proposals for the NHS budget to be incrementally increased in line with changes in the population of the elderly ('this year's plus a bit more'). Abel-Smith's and Titmuss's calculations of the future cost to the NHS of demographic changes (carried out for the Guillebaud Committee, 1956) suggested an increase in total NHS expenditure of 8.1 per cent between 1951–52 and 1971–72. This was equivalent to an average annual increase of about 0.4 per cent. But of the total increase of 8.1 per cent, only around 3.5 per cent was attributable to changes in the population of the elderly, with 4.5 per cent resulting from projected increases in the total population. Abel-Smith and Titmuss made many assumptions in order to arrive at their figures and relied on population projections which turned out to be inaccurate. As Bosanquet and Gray point out, one lesson to be learnt from this is the difficulty of producing reliable predictions of future dependency ratios and hence estimates of future cost pressures on the NHS. Another lesson is the realism of the initial assumptions. Abel-Smith and Titmuss invoked the economist's classic all-embracing assumption of *ceteris paribus* in order to make headway with their calculations. In effect this meant assuming, amongst other things, no change in factors such as the incidence and character of disease; or the quantity and quality of treatment; or the standards of diagnosis; or the present level of unsatisfied demand. Abel-Smith and Titmuss emphasized in their contribution to the Guillebaud Committee that their assumptions were indeed unrealistic, but necessary.

Changes in population size and structure seem self-evidently important factors to take into account in any budget-setting exercise. But there are other factors related to the demand for, and supply of, health care. For example, Bosanquet and Gray note that there are significant differences in health-service use according to marital status, as is evident from Figure 4.5. By and large, for all age groups, single people make greater use of the NHS (because they are generally more in need of health care) than either married, widowed or divorced people. The differences can be quite striking:

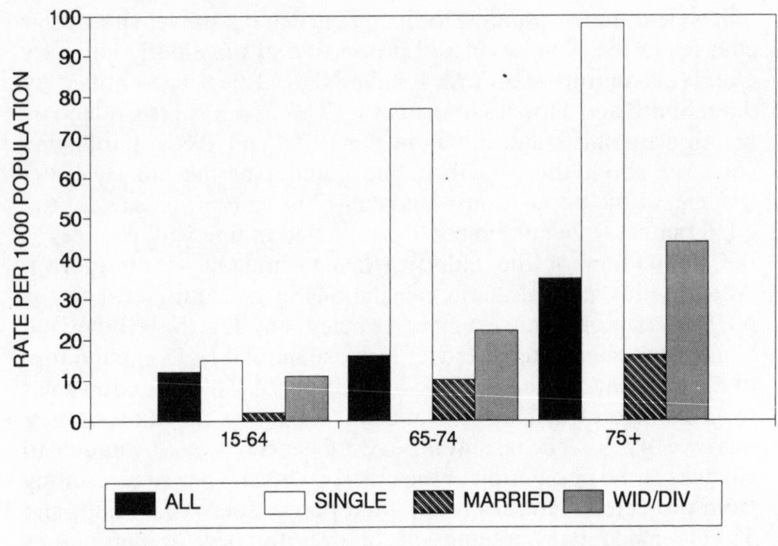

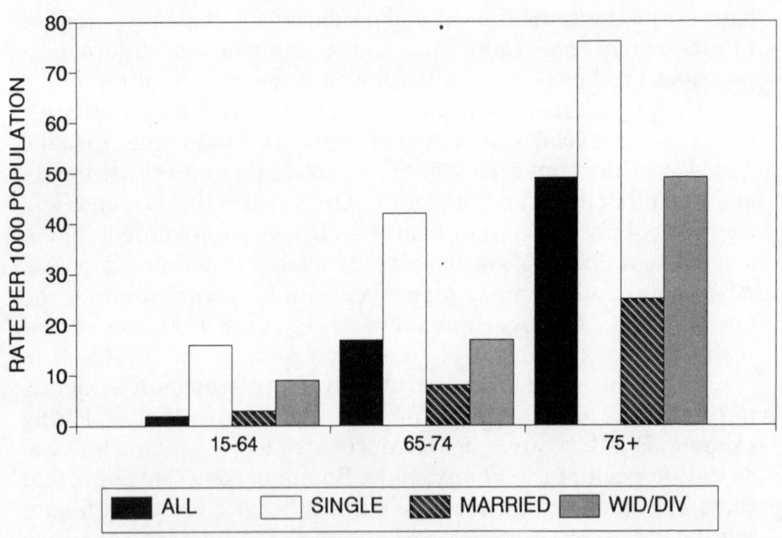

Figure 4.5 In-patient rates per 1000 population (1971): Top, males; bottom, females.

Source: Bosanquet and Gray (1989).

single men aged between 65 and 74 years have in-patient admission rates which are nearly five times the average for their age group, for example. Apart from changes in cultural and social factors affecting the demand for health services, there are significant supply-side pressures as well.

Funding medical advance and technological change

In addition to demographic pressures on NHS expenditure, Maynard and Bosanquet (1986) examined two other strong influences on NHS spending: advances in medicine and the costs of implementing central government health policies. Technological change in medicine is ongoing and unstoppable. And, although it would not be desirable to stop such change, there is a tendency for new treatments and diagnostic procedures to be more expensive than those they replace. Some new procedures are brand new, opening up new areas of medicine and creating new levels of demand by their mere existence/discovery. Advances in medicine are very hard to resist even if, judged by economic and even effectiveness criteria, they would appear not worth doing. There are many examples of medical advances and new surgical techniques which, in their infancy, were heavily criticized both on economic and effectiveness grounds but which have been pursued (largely by clinicians) to the point where they have become accepted. Heart transplant surgery is such a case which, through improved knowledge and technique, has continually increased its effectiveness and efficiency. Arguments against such surgery have now switched to criticism of heart transplants for babies, in line with improvements in the outcome of surgery for adults and the extension by clinicians of this technique to younger and younger patients.

Estimates of the effects of medical advance on expenditure are difficult to make. The Department of Health's estimate of an annual increase in expenditure needed to cope with medical advance of 0.5 per cent of the total hospital and community health service (HCHS) budget (equivalent to about £80 m. in 1991–92) includes broad assumptions about, for example, levels of throughput, efficiency and unit costs. The methodology used by the Department to arrive at a figure of 0.5 per cent is not based on close monitoring of the extra costs of specific medical advances, but rather on a broad-brush approach which analyses past trends in the number of acute cases and their costs (Maynard and Bosanquet, 1986; Harrison and Gretton, 1986).

Whilst these assumptions and methodology can be easily criticized, there is perhaps a more fundamental criticism based on the apparently implicit assumption that, in effect, all medical advance must be accepted and hence funded. In fact, Maynard and Bosanquet, as economists, would not accept this assumption and would argue that all new medical advances need to be rigorously examined for their economic and medical effectiveness before they are taken on by the NHS to become mainstream services. The problem is that such examination either does not take place at all, or is inadequately carried out. On a pragmatic level, however, the fact is that new medical techniques keep occurring, with the consequent pressure from clinicians (and very often patients) for these techniques to be used. Preventing new medical techniques being used because of inadequate medical evidence of their effectiveness is hard in the face of such pressure; to do so on the grounds of inadequate evidence of economic effectiveness is even harder. These criticisms touch on the fundamental criticism of the incremental approach to global NHS budget setting, and it is really a criticism of the degree to which one accepts the pragmatism involved in arriving at an answer to the question which must have an answer – how much should the NHS spend next year, the year after and the year after that?

Funding health policy changes

The second factor which Maynard and Bosanquet note is the question of funding the direct and indirect resource consequences of government policies. As with medical advance, costing these resource consequences is somewhat imprecise. Maynard and Bosanquet list various factors such as tackling AIDS, deinstitutionalization and the move to community care, health promotion, etc. which they have identified as contributing to cost pressures in the NHS and, economic evaluation of their worth apart, need to be included in any incremental budget calculation. Whilst Maynard and Bosanquet do not give an overall figure for the likely cost of funding policy initiatives, an annual increase of 0.5 per cent has become conventional wisdom. Aside from the lack of any significant methodology, the same basic problem still arises of the

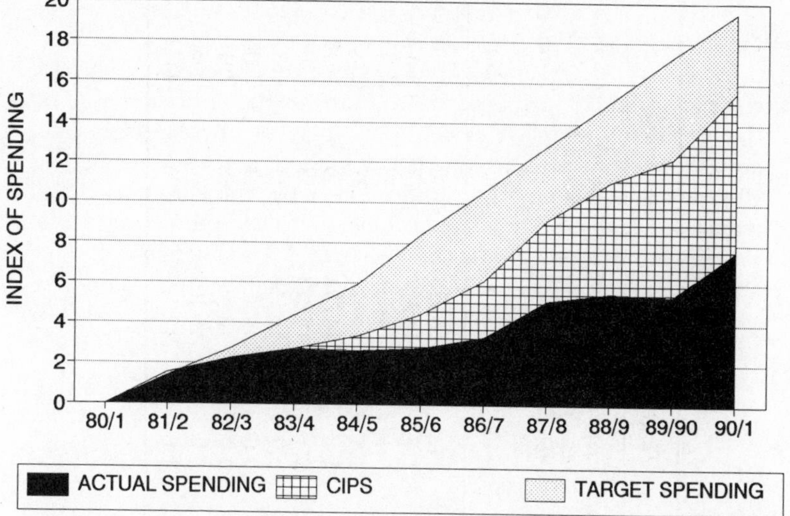

Figure 4.6 Target and actual funding 1980/1–1990/1, hospital and community health service, England (1990–91 prices). CIPS = Cost-improvement programmes.

Source: NAHAT (1990b).

acceptability of the pragmatism involved in arriving at a figure of 0.5 per cent as arose with the estimates of the costs of medical advance.

Underfunding

Bearing in mind the problem of the acceptability of the pragmatic approach to NHS funding levels, what kind of picture of NHS expenditure is obtained if the various elements of this approach are brought together and applied to actual expenditure levels? Table 4.1 and Figure 4.6 show actual and target funding for the English HCHS taking account of demographic change, medical advance and central Government health policies between 1980–81 and 1990–91. These figures come from the National Association of Health Authorities and Trusts (NAHAT, 1990b) and are similar to other calculations carried out by other groups (for example, King's Fund Institute, 1988). What these figures show is that, even allowing for efficiency gains (cost improvement savings being used

Table 4.1 Calculating underfunding for the English hospital and community health services (HCHS): 1980–81

Year	*Actual spending*			*Spending + savings*		*'Target' spending*		*Underfunding*	
	Cash allocation	*HCHS inflation*	*Allocation at 1990–91 prices*	*Recurrent CIPS**	*Allocation + CIPS 1990–91 prices*	*Required real increase*	*'Target' spending*	*Annual shortfall*	*Cumulative under-funding*
	(£m.)	*(%)*	*(£m.)*	*(£m.)*	*(£m.)*	*(%)*	*(£m.)*	*(£m.)*	*(£m.)*
1980–81	6 999	–	14 025	0	14 025	–	14 025	0	0
1981–82	7 688	8.2	14 239	0	14 239	1.4	14 222	–17	–17
1982–83	8 251	6.5	14 349	0	14 349	1.4	14 421	72	55
1983–84	8 709	5.1	14 410	0	14 410	1.5	14 637	227	283
1984–85	9 208	5.8	14 401	105	14 506	1.6	14 871	366	648
1985–86	9 699	5.2	14 419	237	14 656	2.3	15 213	558	1206
1986–87	10 421	6.9	14 492	395	14 887	2.0	15 518	631	1837
1987–88	11 507	8.5	14 749	568	15 317	2.0	15 828	511	2348
1988–89	12 758	10.5	14 798	778	15 576	2.0	16 145	568	2916
1989–90	13 765	8.0	14 784	964	15 748	2.0	16 467	720	3636
1990–91	15 099	7.4	15 099	1114	16 213	1.8	17 019	806	4442

Source: NAHAT (1990b)

* CIPS = Cost improvement programmes

as a proxy for such gains), there has been a gap between what should have been spent on the English HCHS and what was actually spent.

Although these are calculations based on historic expenditure data, the 'target' line can be extended into future years (as it is in Figure 4.6) by drawing on population projections and assuming constant increases in expenditure of 0.5 per cent to fund medical advance and central Government health policies.

LAST YEAR PLUS A BIT MORE – IF WE CAN AFFORD IT

Although in essence the incremental approach to funding levels described above is the broad approach used by government (see, for example, cmd 484 Social Services Committee Memorandum of Evidence from the Department of Health, House of Commons, 1990) one particular criticism of this funding methodology was that, politically, governments could not abrogate their financial control of public spending to what appeared to be a formula which contained no limits. That is, the formula suggested ever increasing amounts of money to be spent on the NHS, eating up more and more of the nation's wealth, without regard to affordability.

A 1987 report by O'Higgins on behalf of the Institute of Health Services Management, the British Medical Association and the Royal College of Nursing (1987) tried to overcome the affordability criticism by linking a version of the incremental approach to a measure reflecting the nation's wealth – in this case the gross domestic product (GDP). O'Higgins' proposal was not simply a matter of linkage to some affordability criteria, but also attempted to resolve other issues related to funding levels of a state-financed health-care system. For instance, the proposal tried to allow for growth in the real pay of NHS staff (most of whom have seen their comparative real pay levels fall for many years). In doing so, however, it recognized a trade off between pay and service levels.

Calculations using this GDP method showed that actual NHS spending in 1987–88 was some £172 m. short. In 1988–89 it was £602 m. short, and by 1989–90 had fallen to £916 m. below the target growth implied by the GDP arithmetic. By 1989–90 cumulative shortfalls over just three years were £1690 m. – just over 9 per cent of the total budget.

Clearly, there seem to be two major criticisms of this approach.

The first is the question of what happens when GDP is falling or, at least, only rising marginally? It is at such times, when economic activity is low or when the economy is in recession, that health-care demand tends to rise (through the effects of unemployment, lower pay, etc.). This suggests that there perhaps needs to be an inverse relationship between GDP and health-care funding. Or, on the other hand, that there should be a minimum baseline growth. But this negates the reason for the GDP linkage in the first place. The second criticism echoes the criticism of the straightforward incremental approach, which is that no government is likely to willingly surrender their control of a significant slice of public expenditure to a formula dictating spending levels. Whether this is a valid position for a government to hold can be questioned, of course, particularly if public pressure to maintain spending on the NHS is significant (which it appears to be). Nevertheless, if the GDP approach is trying to find a practical or pragmatic solution to the thorny problem of health-care funding levels then it needs to be pragmatic enough to overcome this political problem, which it seems not to be.

Finally, O'Higgins' proposal does not distinguish between public and private provision of health care, treating them as one homogeneous lump. The implication of this is that there can be a trade off between public and private provision. But this ignores the distributional issues that could arise from such a trade off, or the desirability of the private sector crowding out parts of the public sector and the effects this could have on the remainder of the public sector and its patients (who are likely to be low income, high health risk and uninsurable).

INTERNATIONAL COMPARISONS

An alternative to the approaches to funding so far described, is to look at how other countries finance their health-care systems, in particular the level of resources they commit to health care. There are many other areas in which international comparisons are used to obtain some sort of picture of how well or badly the UK is performing – from educational attainment and divorce rates to inflation and industry-specific productivity rates – so why not compare health-care systems?

This is not a rhetorical question. There are, in fact, many reasons why comparing the UK's health-care system with other countries' systems is unsatisfactory. Not only is it notoriously difficult to amass comparable data, but interpreting and drawing conclusions from what data can be gathered are highly susceptible to the dismissive criticism that, as Parkin (1989) notes, 'special factors (e.g. cultural) make it [health care] different here (or elsewhere)'. So, even if the right conversions to allow for currency differences and differences in purchasing power within different countries can be made, and even if it can be proved that like is being compared with like in terms of health-care services, it is still not possible to be sure of any conclusions that are drawn.

But the difficulties are not just to do with the variations in statistical systems across countries. Cultural variations of the very notion of what constitutes healthiness or illness, variations in the pattern and structure of disease and the consequent difference in the type of health care supplied, all make straightforward comparison of health-care systems difficult. Moreover, the way health care is supplied and paid for add further complications. Finally, there are serious theoretical problems associated with international comparisons arising from the way economic ideas and interpretations are made and applied (Parkin, McGuire and Yule, 1987).

With this somewhat daunting list of riders and qualifications in mind, and before expanding on some of the problems, it is perhaps useful to detail some of the figures being criticized. Table 4.2 shows health-care expenditure per head using three different methods of comparison. For each method of comparison it can be seen that the spending league table changes. For example, the USA goes from being the highest spender per capita if health-care expenditures are corrected to a comparative base using exchange rates, to the eighth highest spender if international differences in the price of medical care is taken into account (medical care purchasing power parties). The first column is based on exchange rates, i.e. each country's per capita spending is converted to a common currency ($US) according to the relative value of each currency compared with the dollar. The second column converts per capita spending to $US on the basis of GDP purchasing power parities (PPP). PPPs are a statistical construct developed by international bodies such as the Organization for Economic Co-operation and Development (OECD) and the United Nations Statistical Office (UNSO) in an attempt to overcome problems of common conversion using exchange rates (which go up and down for reasons unrelated to such things as a

Table 4.2 Health care expenditures per person for 18 OECD countries, converted by exchange rates and purchasing power parities ($US, 1980)

Country	*Exchange rates*	*(rank)*	*GDP purchasing power parities*	*(rank)*	*Medical care purchasing power parities*	*(rank)*
Norway	964	(5)	773	(6)	1440	(1)
France	1040	(3)	839	(3)	1267	(2)
Netherlands	988	(4)	777	(5)	1168	(3)
Finland	684	(11)	564	(11)	1157	(4)
Austria	722	(10)	607	(9)	1119	(5)
Japan	569	(12)	537	(13)	1118	(6)
Germany	1065	(2)	818	(4)	1108	(7)
USA	1089	(1)	1089	(1)	1089	(8)
Luxembourg	836	(7)	707	(7)	1070	(9)
UK	548	(13)	484	(15)	907	(10)
Belgium	747	(9)	596	(10)	906	(11)
Denmark	880	(6)	668	(8)	894	(12)
Canada	788	(8)	853	(2)	890	(13)
Italy	479	(15)	541	(12)	854	(14)
Ireland	480	(14)	510	(14)	684	(15)
Spain	334	(16)	376	(16)	544	(16)
Portugal	150	(18)	237	(17)	502	(17)
Greece	175	(17)	211	(18)	388	(18)
Average per cap. spending	696		670		952	

Source: Parkin (1989)

Note: For each method of converting per capita spending on health care, the columns denoted 'rank' indicate the highest (1) through to lowest (18) spenders.

country's health-care spending and hence produce converted expenditures which vary over time and which are hard to interpret). GDP PPPs show the cost of health care to an economy as a whole, allowing for differences in the level of *general* prices between countries. Finally, the last column shows spending converted using health-care-specific PPPs. These show the volume of health-care services provided (in monetary terms), allowing for differences in *health-care* prices between countries. This takes account of the fact that in the USA for example, physicians' fees/incomes are generally higher than in, say, the UK. Without taking account of such medical care price differentials any comparison of health-care spending is meaningless.

Whilst the USA slips from being the highest spender to being the eighth highest (depending on the conversion methods used) the UK improves its position from thirteenth to tenth if medical care prices are taken into account and not just exchange rate differences. Another way of looking at Table 4.2 is to compare the UK's position against an *average* per capita spending for each of the three conversion methods. Average spending per head is shown at the bottom of the table. On the basis of exchange rate conversion and GDP purchasing power parties, the UK is 27 per cent and 28 per cent *below* the average. But when medical care purchasing power parties are used, the UK is only 5 per cent below average *per capita* spending.

How, in the context of budget setting for the NHS, can this information be used? Superficially the figures suggest that too little is spent. But if that is the case how much should be spent: the average? Twice the average? The most? The average of which spending figure, those based on exchange rates, those based on GDP PPPs, those based on medical care PPPs?

Rather than make what must be an arbitrary choice concerning where the UK should lie in these rankings, an alternative, and perhaps less arbitrary choice could be based on the apparent relationship between the wealth of a country and the amount of that wealth it devotes to health care. In part, it was this correlation which informed the GDP-linked incremental spending proposals of O'Higgins. Chapter 3 showed that the links between a country's wealth and health-care spending (as measured by per capita expenditure) were found to be strongly positive, suggesting that, for example, an increase in GDP of 10 per cent leads to an increase in health-care spending of more than 10 per cent (most studies agree on a figure of around 13 per cent, in fact). This, in turn, has led many to claim that health care is an economic luxury and not the necessity one may have presumed. (It should be noted that the terms 'luxury' and 'necessity' are used in their economic context and relate to calculations of income elasticity.) But it is clear from Parkin *et al.* (1987) that these associations depend crucially on the data used, the conversion methodology and on the application of the correct economic theory in order to interpret the association. In fact, many of the conclusions drawn from the association between GDP and per capita health-care spending are changed or even overturned if, instead of using exchange rates to convert different countries' health-care spending to a common unit, purchasing power parities are used. Firstly, the association becomes weaker, and secondly, the UK appears to spend about the right amount on health care given its wealth, but pays less than average for it. This is in contrast to other studies (King's Fund Institute, 1988) which have suggested that the UK spends up to 30 per cent less than its GDP suggests it should.

The tremendous difficulties inherent in the exercise of comparing health-care systems across countries would appear to render such exercise less than useful in the context of gaining some practical handle on the vexed question of the right level of funding for the UK's health-care system.

VOTING ON VALUES

The value issue is, as Parkin (1989) points out, a normative one. And as such, is a question which is not readily amenable to the sorts of analyses so far discussed. All these approaches depend on appeals to the facts to build some sort of argument about what funding levels should be. Apart from the disagreements that arise over which facts are really 'facts' and how these should then be interpreted, the very tools being used are wrong. It is like trying to be objective about something that is inherently subjective. It is the difference between the economists' notion of positive and normative (assertions, statements, hypotheses, etc.). The preceding analyses are more appropriately linked with statements about what funding levels will be rather than what they ought to be. The former implies that the analyses can be disproved in the sense that their predictions turn out to be wrong. But the latter removes the issue from such scientific scrutiny and lodges it firmly in the realm of value judgements and hence neither provable nor disprovable by reference to 'the facts'. But if the question/answer is now reduced to 'we spend/fund what we want to spend/fund', does this leave us any the wiser? It does and it does not. In one sense, it clarifies the issue by pointing up the value judgements involved in solving the question. On the other hand, this still does not help formulate a practical solution to the question.

However, there is, in a democracy, a well known way of resolving difficult issues involving value judgements. It is called voting. In theory, the difficulties referred to earlier about trade offs at national level between, say, education and health care, and more generally the values attached to different priorities concerning the use of limited resources can be resolved by letting society (i.e. all of us) express its collective opinion through some form of voting system. To some extent this is done already. Through general and local elections the electorate nominate individuals/groups to put into action manifestos on its behalf.

Despite the checks and balances within most democratic systems, politicians, once elected, are not irrevocably bound to their manifesto pledges. The current reforms of the NHS are a classic example of a major political initiative which did not even appear in any manifesto. Apart from the fact that politicians have a representative, not mandated role, there arise questions as to what is being voted for and who is doing the voting. In national elections what is being voted for is a broad package of policies dealing with many aspects of public and private life, not just health care. It could be argued that this is no bad thing as it forces society to make just those sorts of trade offs which involve value judgements and which are nigh on impossible to solve using the 'positive' approaches detailed earlier on. The system, however, is not perfect. Arrayed before the voters at election time is only a very small fraction of all the possible combinations and permutations of policies governments could adopt. In effect, the electorate faces a very limited choice, and it can quite possibly turn out to be the case that on the specific issue of health care the party elected to power do not represent the broad will of the electors (although on other issues they do).

The question of who votes is very important in the context in which this issue is being discussed. Currently there are various groups in the community who are excluded from voting in national or local elections: peers of the realm, convicts, anyone aged under 18 years and patients in mental institutions are perhaps the main groups. All of these groups make use of the NHS in some form or other. In particular, the last two groups make significant use of the NHS. Accepting the reasons for their disenfranchisement, what are the ethics of a system which makes decisions (in this case, decisions about health-care funding) affecting someone's life but excludes them from the primary decision-making process of voting? There is a parallel here with the notion of 'no taxation without representation'. In this case it might be, 'no spending of taxes without representation'. Apart from those specifically excluded from voting there are many who do not vote or find it difficult to vote, not only for political reasons, but because they are unable to do so. Again, what are the ethics of a voting system which potentially discriminates against important users of the health-care services such as the housebound infirm elderly?

It is, of course, all too easy to criticize a system of voting and political organization designed, not to generate an answer to the highly specific problem of the appropriate level of health-care funding every year, but to arrive at a broad consensus of the way a nation would like its government to tackle a whole range of issues that are generally felt to be best done by governments and not left to individuals. And if this includes electing a government which has the view that some things are in fact best left (or given back) to individuals to do, then this reveals, perhaps, one of the strengths of the system (whether or not one agrees with such a view).

Apart from opinion poll evidence which almost always indicates that people want more spent on the health services (even if this means higher taxes), there are few examples of the issue of health-care funding being the subject of a systematic community-wide vote or ballot designed to have specific and direct influence over funding levels. However, there has been a related experiment concerning the prioritization of health-care activities which exhibited many of the problems that would be encountered with such a way of dealing with the question of funding levels. The experiment took place in the USA, in Oregon, in 1989, and involved the state's electorate voting on an ordering of around 2000 medical services priorities within the Medicaid program (an insurance system covering people on low incomes). In terms of holding any lessons for the NHS, the Oregon experiment has been criticized as a product of the specific cultural, political and medical system environment of Oregon in particular and the USA generally (Klein, 1991). Whilst it is undoubtedly true, as Klein says, that the experiment is anchored in Oregon's political system, two issues that have been highlighted by the experiment are, on the one hand, the need for information on the part of the electorate to enable them to vote sensibly (e.g. information about properly evaluated outcomes of care) and on the other, those inseparable components of voting, namely, argument, persuasion and dialogue. Klein lays emphasis on these later corollaries of voting, but it must surely be the case that argument, persuasion and dialogue can only sensibly take place if they are informed by hard data about, for example, the outcome of medical intervention, which often have the merit of clarifying the value judgements that require argument, persuasion and dialogue.

A rather macabre analogy is the issue of capital punishment. Part of the explanation for Members of Parliament consistently not voting for its return; whilst public opinion polls show unwaivering support for the idea is the former's consideration of the hard evidence that the only people for which capital punishment truly acts as a deterrent are those who have been executed. The rest of the explanation of the difference between MPs and the public lies in the views MPs take about the value judgements involved in the issue – such as retributive justice and state-sanctioned revenge. The point is that whilst the question of whether or not capital punishment should be reintroduced cannot be solved entirely by recourse to the evidence on its effectiveness as a deterrence, knowledge of that information exposes the real issues that are legitimately a matter for argument, etc.

It is the case, however, that one very important piece of information required to inform the debate about health-care funding – outcome measures – also needs a hefty input of value judgements if they are to be useful. Measures of the outcome of medical intervention such as quality-adjusted life years (QALYs) need agreement about 'quality' and about the ordering of different health states. Reaching community-wide agreement on the value judgements involved would be an enormous task. But it is only after such agreement that the value judgements involved in the issue of health-care funding can then be properly addressed through argument, persuasion, dialogue and ultimately, voting. Clearly, if, as Klein argues, QALYs are not a quick technological fix, neither is voting and its associated democratic activities a quick political fix.

As with the other approaches to the question of health-care funding, the acceptability of the democratic stategy hinges on the degree of imperfection one is willing to put up with in order to avoid the paralysis of not reaching some sort of answer.

CONCLUSION

If there are two points to be drawn from this brief review of approaches to NHS funding levels it is that in an imperfect world with imperfect information, imperfect solutions are the norm, and that it is vital to separate (the disprovable) facts from (the unprovable) value judgements. But moreover, it is clear that it is only in tackling *both* the 'facts' *and* the 'value judgements' that an answer to 'how much of our scarce resources do we commit to the NHS?' can be properly formulated. For the foreseeable future the task for policymakers, government and all involved in this funding decision is to improve on the quality and quantity of the data available to inform this funding decision and also to improve the systems currently used to deal with the value judgements the vexed question of funding necessarily embodies.

5

A MARKET FOR HEALTH CARE

Chapter 4 looked at various ways that the question 'how much do we spend on health care?' could be tackled from a pragmatic point of view, i.e. recognizing that the information and the decision systems needed to answer the question in an ideal way are inadequate. The extent to which the information set needed over the next decade will be improved is open to speculation. This is also true for improvements in the way value judgements involved in answering the funding question are dealt with. Improvements are speculative partly due to technical problems involved, and partly due to an uncertainty concerning the will to further tackle the difficult issues that necessarily arise – issues that include the hegemony of the medical profession, making explicit the trade offs that have to be made between competing commitments on scarce resources and so on.

Alluded to at the beginning of Chapter 4, however, was a possible solution to the problem of funding – to privatize the decision. In other words, to let individuals directly decide themselves what they want to spend on health care – health care for themselves. Why not treat health care like most other goods and services in a capitalist economy: as something to buy if wanted, and can be afforded?

Whilst most of the indications are that health care in the UK is not on the verge of a transformation into a full-bloodied market, there should be no presumption that there will be no development or expansion of limited market-type systems in health care in the near future. This is not just because of the obvious fact that the reforms of the NHS have already set up a pseudo market, but also because there are historical trends, supplemented by deliberate policies, which suggest an expansion in the private, market-based, health-care sector.

The main intention of this chapter is to examine the financial issues arising from the treatment of health care as a market commodity. What will become clear is that, in practice, markets not only tend to produce outcomes which are thought generally undesirable (and which have led to extensive state intervention in an attempt at correction) but also, through the financing mechanisms markets have developed (for example, insurance) and the way these have been organized, that markets have also created problems for themselves (leading to, for example, various forms of merger between the organizations who pay for health care and those who provide it).

A MARKET – BUT WHAT KIND?

Markets do not have a simple, unique identity but exist in many different forms, involving varying degrees of freedom, price and other statutory regulation. This last 'interference' in the market can include direct interventions by government to control output, quality, who is allowed to sell and who is allowed to buy. But although markets can vary according to the extent of regulation, and although this – and barriers to entry of markets by potential producers, creating disparate market types with apparently unique characteristics – the difference between a health-care system dominated by state funding and provision and a health-care market must be the extent to which prices are used as a guide to exchange in the latter, and non-price criteria, such as need, are used as a guide to distribution in the former.

The overt notion of the NHS is the explicit rebuttal of the use of prices as a means of determining how health care is distributed. Although the alternative allocation criteria of 'need' has evaded determined attempts at an agreed definition, there is at least a consensus that it does not include any notion of discrimination on non-health grounds. And, amongst other things, these include the means (or income) of users and the cost (or price) of their treatment/care. Of course, given that it is funded from taxes which overall are generally progressive, the NHS does discriminate on the grounds of income. But this discrimination is really just a perverse way of looking at redistribution (in kind) from the wealthy (in the form of taxation) to the less wealthy (in the form of health care). It is arguable whether the NHS has managed to live up to this redistributive ideal. But nevertheless, in the context of this discussion, it is useful to define a market in health care as a system which does, unlike the NHS, discriminate on the grounds of income (but this time in the sense that the well-off can afford to buy more health care than the less well-off) and price (in the sense that consumers of health care more directly bear the costs of their own consumption of health care).

Other characteristics of the market that may be prespecified will of course include the differentiation between buyers or purchasers of care on the one hand, and sellers or providers of care on the other. Questions of ownership, structure and form of the market are more difficult to answer in the abstract as many possibilities exist. There is probably a line of enquiry here of the form 'when is a market not a market?' or, was (is?) the NHS just a special form of market involving a monopolist and a monopsonist who are one and the same?

However, in the abstract there is probably not much more that needs to be said about markets other than the fact that there are buyers, sellers and a mechanism (prices) to equate the former's demand with the latter's supply. In practice, however, it is the way the particular ABC economy for health care has developed and been forced to move on from this simple notion of exchange which is of real interest.

FINANCING: INSURANCE

It is evident that where health-care markets exist, financing is not only by the usual methods of direct payment by consumers (as with most goods and services in market-orientated economies) but also indirect payment through insurance. The reason for this is the particular combination of the uncertainty of the occurrence of illness and the form, amount and costs of health care that will be needed as a result. Singly, uncertainty of occurrence, form, amount and cost are not sufficient characteristics to necessarily justify insurance. Just because an individual cannot accurately predict when they will need to replace some item of clothing ruined by their mis-programmed washing machine, does not mean that they automatically purchase 'washing insurance'. Whilst presumably there are some people who may want (or have even tried) to negotiate premiums for such an insurance, generally the demand is low, as is the willingness of any insurer to take on the risk at a premium level the insured can afford. In principle, therefore, although the costs of uncertain events can be insured, whether or not there is significant demand for, and supply of, insurance depends on a range of factors.

For health care, as for other goods and services with similar characteristics, insurance offers a way of spreading risk, in this case the risk of paying medical care bills. In return for a premium (based on some kind of assessment of likely future occurrence of illness and hence health-care costs) an insurer will take on the burden of risk. In order for premiums to be set at a reasonable level for individuals (and for insurers to stay in business) insurance companies need to attain a balance of risks held to likely payout. Given that insurance companies cannot predict with accuracy the risks for every individual they insure, the easiest way to achieve this balance is to attract a reasonably large, random number of customers. In this way the insurance company will maximize the chances of balancing good risks with bad and hence not find themselves going out of business. The difficulties that insurers and insured alike face from problems such as 'adverse selection' and 'moral hazard' are discussed below.

Whilst insurance undoubtedly allows more people to gain access to health care than would otherwise be the case if the only form of financing was the direct payment of the full costs of health care at the time they were consumed, consumers' costs (in terms of insurance premiums), although reduced, are not zero and therefore variations in access still remain. Conversely, insurance can create problems of overconsumption and spiralling provider costs when, as has typically been the case, insurers have lacked any incentives to increase their negligible control over providers' financial management. These problems, some of the related responses of the insurance market and some of the governmental policies which have been introduced to deal with the perceived failings of health-care markets, take up the remainder of this chapter.

Rationing

In the USA, which, at 60 per cent of total expenditure, has the highest percentage of private financing (approximately 33 per cent direct payments and 28 per cent from insurance premiums) of health care of any major industrialized country, over 37 million people (including 10 million children) are uninsured. Millions more have inadequate insurance (Reinhardt, 1991). In the absence of insurance, many more people would find it impossible to pay for the health care they needed. Nevertheless, there is an increasing concern in the USA that one of the richest nations in the world, with some of the most sophisticated health-care technologies in the world, ends up in the 1990s with a system of health-care financing which effectively denies access to health care to nearly 20 per cent of its population. These problems are now being addressed by the new Clinton Administration.

One consequence of privatizing the health-care funding decision is that individuals may decide either to underinvest in health care (not buy enough medical insurance to cover their need for health care, for example) or not invest at all. Whilst this suggests that health care is not the necessity that might be presumed (that is, in the economist's sense, that demand for health-care insurance does not vary with a person's income – i.e. demand is inelastic with respect to income), such interpretations need to be handled with care. A more obvious explanation of a decision not to buy insurance is that the 'decision' is not a free choice, but one forced on an individual through low income or a straightforward bar on insurance purchase because they are considered a 'bad risk'. The use of terms such as 'necessity' and its counterpart, 'luxury', given these circumstances is misleading. The reality of medical insurance as experienced in the USA, for example, is that low income and bad risk are significant factors affecting the take up of insurance. For many millions of Americans on low incomes, the effective 'choice' is between paying medical insurance bills now, to cover for an event which will occur some time in the future, and paying for immediate needs such as food and housing. The trade off is between a cost which will occur in the future (the costs of treatment, etc.) and costs which occur now, in the present (the costs of food, etc.).

Adverse selection

The problem of the inability to pay for medical insurance can be compounded by another problem associated with imperfections or asymmetries in the information available in the insurance market. Because consumers of insurance tend to have a better estimate of their own probability of needing health care than insurers, and because premiums are set on the basis of insurers' knowledge of the general probabilities of consumption, there will be some individuals for whom the cost of premiums outweigh the direct costs of future health-care treatment. Although the future costs of treatment are likely to be greater than the costs of regular premium payments, because the former occur some time in the future, their value is diminished when compared to the more certain and regular payments of premiums. Those people who estimate that their premium costs outweigh their future health-care costs may feel it is not worth insuring. Conversely, for others, insurance premiums may be, in their estimation, good value for money, and so they insure. The outcome for insurers is a potential increase in 'bad risks' and losses of income as premiums increasingly fail to cover payouts to claimants. This adverse selection can, if left to itself, completely destroy the insurance market: with increased payouts insurers increase their income (i.e. raise premiums), but this merely leads to more people opting out of insurance and deciding to self-insure. The problem of rising premium prices is compounded.

As noted earlier, insurers try and get round the problem of rising premium prices by increasing the pool of insured persons: for example, by linking insurance plans to employee groups. This is essentially a form of compulsory insurance. Insurers also try to improve their knowledge of individuals' health-care probabilities, tailoring premiums more directly to each individual's characteristics (hence the increased premiums paid by smokers, for example). Premiums are thus more related to experience than the more generalized knowledge of community-wide probabilities. In addition, insurers restrict the amount of cover they are willing to offer, and introduce 'deductibles' to offset some proportion of payouts. (A deductible is usually an agreed commitment on the part of the insured to pay the first £*x* of any treatment, and is similar to deductibles in other forms of insurance such as for motor cars.) As Culyer (1989) has noted however,

> Though more efficient from a welfarist perspective . . . experience-rating is likely to violate the usual distributional criteria of equity: those with a history of sickness will face the highest premiums, have less comprehensive cover, be most likely to pay deductibles . . . and, since ill-health and income are correlated, will on average be the poorer members of the community.

Culyer's point about equity is important and is discussed further below.

Equity in access/utilization and finance

The US experience suggests that in a market-dominated health-care system, where insurance and direct payments are the main methods of financing, there is significant inequality of access to, and utilization of health care. This is not necessarily to suggest that all the uninsured receive no health care whatsoever, but that, depending on individuals' incomes and health states, there is considerable variation in the quantity and quality of health care to which individuals are able to gain access. The particular equity issue being expressed here is one of *horizontal equity* – that those in equal need receive equal treatment. Judging by the number of uninsured and underinsured this is self-evidently not the case in the USA. Although there are a number of factors which contribute to this situation (discrimination on the grounds of race, variations in geographical access, etc.), the main factor would appear to be the predominant financing methods which inherently discriminate on the grounds of income or ability to pay.

Embedded in these access/utilization issues of health-care equity is also that of the equity concerning the financing of health care. For example, to what extent do actual payments for health care in a system where payments are made either directly or via medical insurance, reflect ability to pay? In a study of equity between health-care systems, Wagstaff, Van Doorslaer and Paci (1989) looked at three countries – the USA, UK and Netherlands – and compared the proportion of total pre-tax income (their measure of ability to pay) for each decile (tenth) of the population with the equivalent deciles' payments for health care. Overall, they found that the USA had a generally regressive system of health-care finance (that is, lower income groups contributed more to total health-care payments than their proportion of total pre-tax income, and vice versa for higher income groups); the Dutch also had a regressive system of health-care finance, but less marked than the USA; and the UK health-care system was, overall, mildly progressive, with the distribution of health-care payments almost exactly matching the distribution of pre-tax income. Wagstaff *et al.* also disaggregated the various forms of finance that exist in each of these countries and found, as Table 5.1 illustrates, health-care financing from direct payments in the USA are very regressive, as are payments via private medical insurance. There are similar findings for The Netherlands with respect to insurance although not for direct

Table 5.1 Measuring the degree of equity of different methods of financing health care

<table>
<tr><th rowspan="2">Country</th><th rowspan="2">Overall measure of progressivity</th><th colspan="5">Index of progressivity for component sources of finance</th></tr>
<tr><th>Income tax</th><th>Pay roll tax</th><th>Direct payments</th><th>Private insurance</th><th>Social insurance</th></tr>
<tr><td>USA</td><td>−0.15</td><td>+0.15</td><td>−0.04</td><td>−0.39</td><td>−0.19</td><td>–</td></tr>
<tr><td>Netherlands</td><td>−0.06</td><td>–</td><td>–</td><td>+0.12</td><td colspan="2">−0.1</td></tr>
<tr><td>UK</td><td>+0.03</td><td>+0.02</td><td>–</td><td>–</td><td>–</td><td>+0.03</td></tr>
</table>

Source: Wagstaff *et al.* (1989)

Notes: The figures are Kakwani's Progressivity Index (KPI). KPI can take values ranging from −2 to +1. KPI <1 implies that the financing method/system is regressive, i.e. the poor's share of health-care financing is greater than their share of total pre-tax income (and vice versa for the rich). KPI >1 implies that the financing method/system is progressive, i.e. the poor contribute proportionately less of their share of pre-tax income to health care, and the rich proportionately more.

payments. Direct payments in The Netherlands in fact only constitute about 4 per cent of total health-care spending (compared with 32 per cent in the USA) and reflect the fact that high income groups often elect to reduce their private insurance premiums by accepting deductibles (i.e. direct payment of part of any insurance claim).

An important point to note, however, is that a progressive health-care system in financing terms does not automatically imply a progressive system in terms of treatment or consumption of health care. The rich may contribute more than the poor to health care, but they may also take out more than would perhaps be deemed equitable as far as their health status is concerned. The obverse of this is that, in terms of their pre-tax income, the poor may be favoured in a progressive system by paying less than their income suggests that they should, but in terms of their health status they may receive less than their fair share of health care. There is some evidence to suggest that this is indeed the case with regard to the NHS (Hurst, 1985). Clearly, there are many factors at work apart from the method of financing which affect the degree of equality with which health care is delivered. Moreover, the main concern is not just with equity on the financing or delivery sides, but with both.

Unlike the definition of equity referred to when considering access/utilization of health care, the particular notion of equity Wagstaff *et al.* investigated on the financing side was *vertical equity*

– that unequals (in terms of ability to pay) are treated unequally. In fact both concepts of equity, horizontal and vertical, are of interest, both on the access/utilization side of health care and on its finance side. However, if these definitions of equity were to be prioritized, the tendency would be to attach more weight to equal treatment for equal need (horizontal equity) on the access/utilization side, and unequal payments for unequal income (vertical equity) on the financing side. It should be noted that whilst studies such as Wagstaff *et al.* have been able to produce some useful evidence concerning equity in different health-care systems, these studies face difficult problems over definitions and particularly quantification/measurement of concepts such as 'access', 'utilization', and, indeed, equity itself.

Nevertheless, what empirical evidence there is tends to support the *a priori* view that the experience of market systems of health-care financing, which, by definition, equate demand and supply through the use of prices (generally for medical insurance as far as users/patients are concerned) result in variations in the levels of consumption of health care which are independent of the need for health care. Unlike most other goods and services in a market economy which exhibit similar variations in consumption however, the response to the experience concerning health care is always some degree of intervention in the market so that access to health care is improved. In the USA, for example, the response to this particular 'failure' of the health-care market has been to set up state-run and state-funded insurance schemes for those on low incomes. In addition, charitable hospitals fill some gaps by providing free or very low cost care. The response in other countries such as the UK has been state intervention on a much greater scale. In The Netherlands the insurance system combines compulsory contributions with private insurance based on risk (often age-related), together with mixtures of employer and employee contributions.

Caring about health

Policies designed to intervene in, or supplement or supplant the market highlight some fundamental attitudes to health and health care. Most economic explanations for the filling of gaps left by health-care markets, or indeed the total substitution of markets by alternative systems of health-care finance and provision, draw on notions and ideas from the 'extra-welfarist' wing of health economics. In essence the extra-welfarist approach relaxes assumptions made by the simply welfarist (that social welfare is a function solely of individual welfare derived only from goods and services directly consumed, for example) and attaches importance to such concepts as caring for others. So, for example, the argument would be, 'not only am I interested in your consumption of health care, such as immunization and vaccination for communicable diseases, because it might affect my health, I am also concerned about your consumption of health care because my welfare or utility (but not necessarily my health) would be adversely affected simply by the pain and distress you might suffer if you consumed too little health care'.

If this seems a convoluted way of stating something rather obvious – the idea that people care about each other – then that is because in some ways it is, but also, it has to be admitted, much is lost in the necessary simplification of the ideas involved. Intervention lends support to the idea of this caring notion with the reason for intervention being the perceived failure of the market to deliver on this principle.

Moral hazard

Whilst the caring principle is important in explaining some of the underlying reasons for intervention in health-care markets which tend to generate a pool of uninsured and underinsured (with consequent underconsumption of health care), there is, paradoxically perhaps, a converse problem associated with insurance which encourages overconsumption and spiralling health-care costs. These particular problems associated with moral hazard have also led to extensive intervention in health-care markets.

Moral hazard can occur with regards to the insured individual and the health-care provider. For example, it can be argued that individuals, once insured, may alter not only their perceptions of risk, but also their actions as a direct result of the fact that they hold insurance. In essence, individuals may become less risk-averse. That is, they may engage in activities – such as smoking – which are harmful to their health but do so because they feel more secure in the knowledge that future costs of treatment are covered by their insurance. As a consequence, there is likely to be an upward pressure on treatment, and hence total health-care costs and, presumably, on premiums, as insurers find payouts exceeding their expectations.

An analogous moral hazard was raised in debates prior to legislation in the UK to make the wearing of car seatbelts compulsory. Opponents of the legislation argued that drivers would feel too secure wearing seatbelts and would tend to be less careful in the way they drove. The importance of this form of moral hazard is hard to adjudge however. Whilst there may be some lowering of risk-aversion due to insurance, health-care costs not only include those direct costs of care (which are covered by insurance) but also the enormous costs of pain, suffering and distress, etc. (which are generally not covered by insurance).

A second form of moral hazard which can potentially arise from insurance is a result of the price-lowering effects insurance brings. At the time of consumption, an insured person faces much reduced health-care costs (which is the main reason to insure in the first place). As a consequence of the lower costs, there is an incentive to increase demand – for example, to seek consultations and possibly treatment which the insured person would not otherwise have done if faced with the full costs of care. As with the previous form of moral hazard, there are off-setting costs involved here which will tend to limit this increase in demand. For example, as with the moral hazard associated with a lowering in risk-aversion, insurance does not cover all the costs associated with health care; individuals still face some substantial, uninsured costs such as travel, time off work, psychic costs related to the process of medical intervention, etc. This last cost may not be negligible. Consider: how actively have you been seeking dental treatment merely because you did not have to pay the full costs of the treatment? Nonetheless, this particular form of moral hazard (which, incidentally, is not limited to health-care systems funded by private insurance but all systems in which there are third-party payers) is thought to lead to significant increases in health-care consumption amongst insured people.

The third form of moral hazard arises on the provider side and has become known as supplier-induced demand, or SID for short (Evans, 1974). As with the informational asymmetries associated with adverse selection, SID is related to the exploitation by doctors of consumers' ignorance about the treatment they need and also the existence of third-party payers (in the shape of the medical-insurance companies). There have been many explanations for the observed positive relationship between health-care utilization and areas in the USA which have high concentrations of physicians. Some explanations involve physicians deliberately exploiting the agency relationship they have with their patients, the fact of third-party paying and the fact that their remuneration was on a fee-per-item basis merely to boost their income or at least maintain it at some target level. Other explanations rely more on the assertion that higher concentrations of physicians lower travel and other health-care-related costs for patients and hence bring out some unmet need (which in turn leads to the observation that physician concentration and health-care utilization are positively related).

Despite the mixed theoretical response to SID, there is empirical evidence which suggests that up to 30 per cent of work in some surgical areas in the USA is inappropriate (Chassim *et al.*, 1987). Again, however, it should be noted that medical variations are not the prerogative of insurance-funded systems, but can be found in all health-care systems (the connection being perhaps the high degree of autonomy exercised by clinicians in all health-care systems). Nevertheless, it is hard to resist the idea that there is some exploitation (mainly of the insurance system rather than the patient) resulting from the particular combination of third-party payers, fee-per-item of service and medical ignorance on the part of patients. Moreover, the notion that doctors do not respond to financial incentives because of some higher ideal based on service to the patient in front of them is not too solidly based; for example, the reluctance of doctors to join the NHS when it was originally set up unless significant pay guarantees were made by the then Ministry of Health up to the sharp increases in immunization and vaccination rates immediately following the system of targets and payment-by-results brought in by the new general practitioner contract in 1990. This suggests at least a passing interest in the pecuniary benefits doctors derive from medicine. Although these examples come from the UK there is nothing to suppose that physicians in the USA behave any differently or that doctors in the UK would behave differently if they worked wholly within a market-based health-care system.

MARKET AND STATE RESPONSES TO MARKET FAILURE

Very broadly, there seem to arise three issues from health-care systems which rely on the private financing decision: unfairness in terms of ability to pay; unfairness in terms of actual access to care; and a lack of incentives to contain costs on the providers' side. Throughout the foregoing on some of the observed 'failures' of market systems of health-care finance, reference has been made to some of the responses these failures have elicited. For example, from the market itself (e.g. the use of deductibles to overcome the problem of overconsumption) and from the state (e.g. the creation of state-run and state-funded insurance schemes to extend coverage to low-income groups). Many of these interventions have proved to be ineffective or counterproductive, failing either to control escalating costs on the one hand or ensure satisfactory quality and/or reduce inequality on the other. Because of the range and sheer number of different interventions that have been tried, no attempt is made here to detail all the permutations and combinations. However, it is interesting to look at the sorts of policies, legislation and reformations that one prime example of a market system of health-care finance, the USA, has undergone in its attempts to deal with the perceived failures of the market.

The list below draws together some of the main state and market responses to market failure. The list is not intended to be comprehensive, but illustrative of the extent to which failure is seen to be a 'bad thing', and the difficulties this failure poses to legislators and others involved in the health-care market.

Responding to market failure: the US experience

Issue	*Response*
Inability to pay for health care	Introduction of medical insurance, e.g. non-profit Blue Shield and Blue Cross in the 1930s
	For-profit medical insurance (1940s)
	Charitable hospitals
	Public hospitals (state funded)

Issue	*Response*
Inability to pay for health care (*cont.*)	'Patient dumping'. Providers cut costs by transferring 'uneconomic' patients to public hospitals. Anti-dumping legislation introduced to prevent transfers on non-medical grounds
Inability to obtain insurance	Federally-funded health-insurance programmes, e.g. Medicaid (for those with low incomes) and Medicare (for those aged over 65 years) (in the 1960s) Compulsory pay-roll taxes in some states to subsidize insurance for those on low incomes (in the 1980s)
Cost inflation	Professional Standards Review Organizations (PSROs) to monitor quality of care and medical necessity of claims made on Medicare and Medicaid PSROs replaced by Peer Review Organizations (PROs) in 1981. PROs given similar remit Cost-sharing policies (e.g. deductibles) to increase burden of health-care costs directly borne by consumers and hence reduce demand pressure on costs Narrowing of definition of medical cover (e.g. certain diagnostic tests not paid for by insurers)

Issue	*Response*
	Tightening of Medicare and Medicaid eligibility rules (65 per cent of low income families covered by Medicaid 10 years ago, now down to 40 per cent) Certificate of Need (CON) introduced by many states to control capital spending by private hospitals and nursing homes (in the 1970s) Encouragement for provider competition following court ruling that 'learned professions' were not exempt from anti-trust laws Combined insurance/provider organizations (e.g. Managed Healthcare Organizations, MHOs, Health Maintenance Organizations, HMOs, etc.) (in the 1960s and 1970s) Preferred Provider Organizations (PPOs). Insurers restrict policyholders to selected providers (in the 1980s) Prospective Payment Systems (PPSs). Replaced Retrospective Payment Systems (RPSs) in the 1980s. Payments set in advance based on predetermined prices for medical procedures (e.g. Diagnosis Related Groups, DRGs)

CONCLUSION

This chapter started with the idea that the seemingly intractable problem of determining the right level of funding for health care could be solved by reasserting consumer sovereignty through the use of markets. However, the market, virtually by definition, produces a 'solution' simply by ignoring certain characteristics which are highly valued and desired – at least judged by the extent of regulation and intervention free health-care markets seem always and everywhere to be subject: that is, some notion of fairness or equity in the way care is financed and delivered. Moreover, the experience of health-care markets in the USA and other countries has been a strong tendency to an inefficient overproduction (through fee-per-item payment systems, non-price competition, etc.) leading to a more costly system for consumers and producers alike.

Markets are of course amoral; this is one of their strengths, enabling complex allocative and productive decisions to be made, with prices guiding buyers and sellers to an equilibrium between demand and supply. This essential amorality of markets is well illustrated by the US economist Mark Pauly (1988) who, in relation to the apparent ineffectiveness of competition in restraining the USA's aggregate health-care spending, argued that increasing the competitiveness of the market would not necessarily lead to lower overall growth in expenditures because this may not be what the consumer wants. The consumer may indeed want higher quality, more expensive health care *even if this is achieved at a cost to others (and in the end to themselves) in terms of higher premiums, inappropriate care, reduced insurance coverage, etc.* In short, the sum of all the sovereign, *amoral* decisions made by consumers can add up to an outcome which many would argue is *immoral*.

Of course, this amoral-to-immoral argument depends on whether, for example, access to health care is seen as a moral issue at all. However, the evidence – the interventionist policies noted throughout this chapter, the existence of socialized forms of health-care systems, etc. – suggests that, for health care, the essential amorality of the 'invisible hand' is seen to be a weakness which leads to patterns of allocation and production which are viewed as failures despite any equilibriating success markets may achieve. In the end, it is a question perhaps of asking markets to do too much: to reconcile objectives such as equity in financing and efficiency of production for which markets are ill-equipped to deal.

6

MANAGING THE MARKET: THE US EXPERIENCE

In looking at market-based mechanisms for financing health care, it is clear from experience (for example, in the USA) that getting the market to produce the right outcome, the desirable outcome as far as equality of access to quality care, fairness in financing and efficiency of production is concerned is not easy. The history of the US health-care system is one of oscillating attempts at regulation and competition. As each new regulatory or competitive structure is raised however, the actors in the market – the physicians, the hospitals, the medical corporations, insurance companies, etc. – find new ways of bypassing the rules, of playing the market game and using the economic incentive structure largely for their own ends. This may seem a harsh summary, but the increasing list of failed policies would suggest that it is not totally unfair.

One question posed in Chapter 5 asked how one of the richest nations in the world can end up with a health-care system which, in the 1990s, despite spending around \$600 bn. on health care (equivalent to nearly three times more per head than in the UK), appears to fail for millions of its citizens? To this could be added that on key health indicators such as infant and perinatal mortality, the US performs exceptionally badly given its per capita GDP (see Table 6.1 and Figure 6.1), and that in the opinion of nearly one-third of the US public, the US health-care system needs to be completely rebuilt (Reinhardt, 1991). This latter finding seems to suggest that the US market-based health care system has significantly failed in one of the market's potentially strongest suits, namely, consumer satisfaction.

One answer to the infant mortality statistic could be that, whilst the USA is a very rich country, it also has great disparity of wealth,

Table 6.1 Selected health status indicators for selected countries

Indicator	*USA*	*UK*	*Germany*	*Nether-lands*	*Japan*	*Canada*
Infant mortality	10.0	9.1	8.3	6.4	5.0	7.9
Perinatal mortality	10.0	8.8	7.3	9.2	6.6	8.4
Male life expectancy	71.5	71.9	71.8	73.5	75.6	73.0
Female life expectancy	78.3	77.6	78.4	80.1	81.4	79.8

Source: OECD (1989)

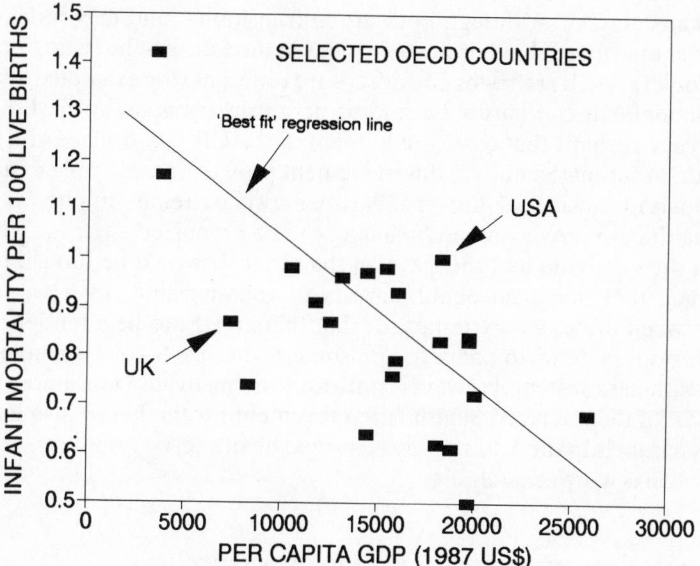

Figure 6.1 Relationship between GDP per head and infant mortality rates.

and low income is strongly correlated with ill health. To expect the health-care system to deal with income inequalities on top of its main job of providing health care may be expecting too much. However, although inequalities in, say, the type of car ownership are not generally thought to merit extensive governmental or other action, inequalities in health and health care *are*, and although the causes of high infant mortality cannot be laid directly at the door of the health-care system (any more than can most other forms of ill health barring, by definition, iatrogenic disease) some attempt at dealing with the problem must be made by the health-care system. This raises the issue of the boundaries of health-care systems – what they are able to do, what they should do, etc.

The main theme in this chapter, however, is the shifts that have been taking place in the US health-care system over the last 20 years, shifts which are taking the system away from a simple market-based way of organizing health care and towards what has been described as a system of managing health-care resources. The parallels between the US and UK health-care systems are by no means perfect. Although both are in transition – and may indeed meet up with each other at some point in the future – the issues and problems each are trying to address are different (for example, cost containment can hardly be said to be a primary issue in the UK, except perhaps that cost containment in the UK is too successful). But, as intimated above, this movement provides an example of an apparent closing of the gap between two extremes in the way health-care provision and financing can be organized – the market on the one hand and the state on the other. It would be foolish to argue that managed health care is the missing link, as it were, between these two extremes, or that there ought to be a tendency for both systems to converge on some form of US-style managed health-care system. However, notwithstanding the obvious importance of the managed health-care movement for the US, it also has its parallels in the UK's newly reformed health service, and for that reason is worth examining.

MANAGED HEALTH CARE: THE MARKET IN TRANSITION?

Although, as Robinson (1990) has noted, to describe the US health-care system as a *system* at all is potentially misleading given the apparent extreme pluralism of the providing and financing institutions. Over the last 20–30 years (and especially over the last decade) there has been some noticeable moves towards what the American Medical Association (AMA) pejoratively called 'socialized medicine'. Such a description goes too far (deliberately so), but it characterized a fear on the part of the medical profession that fee-for-service medicine, from which physicians had benefited, was on its way out, to be replaced by salaries, control, monitoring and effective regulation. In part the AMA were right, for now in the USA, as Weiner and Ferris (1990) have put it, '[Managed health-care organizations, MHOs] are now the modal form of health-care delivery in the US'. Over half of all Americans are now enrolled in one form of managed health-care plan or another, and many other health-care organizations have borrowed ideas and alternative ways of organizing finance and provision from managed health-care organizations such as health maintenance organizations (HMOs).

But what exactly are 'managed health-care organizations'? What are their main characteristics, and how and why have they arisen? Weiner and Ferris cite three main ways that MHOs try to achieve their aims of managing health-care resources (they are not mutually exclusive):

1 A hierarchical vertically-integrated organizational structure.
2 Financial incentives that involve sharing risk with the primary care physician.
3 A series of utilization controls applied to provider practices.

Having noted that there are not always close parallels between the US and UK health-care systems, it should also be noted that there are not always close parallels between US and UK uses of English. So what do these three characteristics mean and how do they distinguish MHOs such as HMOs from traditional financing and providing modes in health care? There is an explanatory problem here, as Weiner and Ferris note when they quote the adage 'When you've seen one HMO . . . you've seen one HMO'. The details of HMOs (and other 'alternative delivery systems' – ADS: or the 'three-letter' health plans as they have become known in the USA) vary tremendously. Weiner and Ferris' three characteristics provide the basic description of HMOs and their offshoots, however.

'Hierarchical vertically-integrated organizational structure' refers essentially to a merger between the financing of health care and its provision. Traditionally, before the emergence of HMOs (or Pre-Paid Group Practices – PPGPs – as they were originally called), the most common health-care model in the USA for the working population was based on private health insurance, generally purchased by employers as an employee benefit. This insurance provided the finance for a system of health-care delivery based on fee-per-item of service, and enabled insured persons to choose the physician/hospital they wanted. By and large, the links between the financing and delivery mechanisms were tenuous to say the least. As was shown in Chapter 5, this tripartite system – where the main business went on between physician and patient, with the financing organization generally following the physician/patient agreement and reimbursing more or less whatever was requested – led to a number of problems, particularly health-care cost inflation. The state/federal health insurance programmes, Medicaid and Medicare, were essentially designed along private sector lines and ran into similar problems. The HMO solution to the problems created by the separation between the financing and providing elements of the system was a vertical integration between the two: the HMO is the insurer and the provider. By this simple expedient the financial incentives in the system are radically altered, with the financing arm of the HMO having a strong financial incentive to take a keen interest in its providing arm.

But the merging of (or at least blurring of the boundaries between) the financing and providing functions implies that the crucial, demand-generating, resource-committing labour component of health care – the physicians – needs to be bound in some way to the ethos of the HMO. HMOs 'lock in' physicians in a number of ways, but mainly through financial incentives based around salaries, budgets or contracts which penalize over-prescription, excessive referral to secondary care, etc. Weiner and Ferris' second distinctive characteristic of HMOs refers to 'sharing risk with the primary care physician'. In essence this means sharing with the HMO the risk that payments by HMO subscribers may be inadequate to cover the costs of care they need. As it is, the primary care physicians control access not only to primary care services they themselves provide (like GPs in the UK) but are also frequently the admitting doctor for hospital care (unlike the UK). With such a set-up there is less incentive to create additional hospital work. The use of salaries (not fee-per-item of service), contracts and budgets also serve to tie the physician into the financial constraints of the HMO.

As well as creating financial incentives for physicians to use resources and manage patients efficiently, HMOs often set up predetermined 'utilization reviews' (particularly with hospitals). Utilization reviews (or URs) aim to reduce unnecessary care, and hence reduce overall costs to the HMO. There are some parallels here with medical audit in the UK, although medical audit is essentially a peer group assessment procedure controlled by clinicians. UR, on the other hand, goes as far as giving the HMO the power to withhold approval for admittance to a hospital if the HMO felt it was not medically justified. (There is a parallel here with the power of District Health Authorities to turn down a request for a non-emergency admission of a patient to a hospital with which the district of residence does not have a contract.) URs also involve retrospective reviews and assessments of discharge criteria, use of tests while patients are in hospital, etc.

It should be clear from this summary of the particular characteristics of HMOs and their offshoots that the central issue they are addressing, or responding to, is that of cost containment. This is not, as has already been said, a problem that immediately springs to mind when considering the UK NHS. Nor can it be said that simply containing costs is the only objective of health-care systems. The ultimate cost containment is achieved when nothing whatsoever is spent. Health-care systems have other aims as well; providing health care is one, and not infringing widely held views about equality (however defined) in health care is another. However, HMOs offer some insights into the use of budgets (cf. GP fundholding), contracts and clinical monitoring, all of which are important constituents of the reformed NHS.

Two further issues require explanation/description before looking at how HMOs have fared in practice and what, if any, lessons could be learned by the NHS. First, there is the question of how HMOs are financed, and second, how they are organized.

Financing HMOs

To all intents and purposes, HMOs are much like any other medical-insurance group. For a fixed, pre-paid sum (a premium), HMOs undertake to ensure access to a specified set of medical services for subscribers. HMOs often offer different packages or policies for different monthly payments. So, rather than tailoring subscriber payments to the individual subscriber (as most insurance policies try to do), they vary the package on offer. In addition, employer-purchased policies are often topped-up by employees to extend coverage to dental and optical care, for instance. Just like any insurance business, HMOs must take cognizance of payments in (the fixed, pre-paid sum) and payments out (expenditure). This is a simple equation which the HMO attempts to manipulate so that the former total more than the latter. One way this can be achieved is to set the right payment level given the expected costs HMOs will incur. There is a restraint, of course, and that is competition. HMOs who set their subscriptions too high risk not attracting enough subscribers to make their business worthwhile. Too low, on the other hand, and the HMO is in the red and heading for bankruptcy. Whilst expanding the 'risk pool' (the greater the number of subscribers, HMOs are better able to predict expenditure based on actuarial formulae) by offering lower subscriptions than others is one tactic, there are other ways of improving expenditure prediction which involve selecting out bad risks. This will be discussed later.

HMOs attempt to adjust both sides of the payments in/payments out equation. As already noted, through the use of various forms of financial incentives and controls over providers, HMOs attempt to reduce the costs of care. If successful, this can feed through to the other side of the equation, allowing lower subscriptions to be set, and consequently increasing the likelihood of attracting more subscribers.

Financing health care by HMOs

Having obtained payments from subscribers, HMOs are then under a contractual obligation to ensure that the future health-care needs of their subscribers are met. In essence, the HMO acts as a purchasing agent on behalf of its subscribers, not actually providing care itself, but ensuring that its customers have access to a pre-specified range of health-care services (cf. the new purchasing role for Health Authorities within the NHS).

In broad terms, HMOs contract with a variety of health-care providers – primary-care physicians, specialists, hospitals, pharmacies, etc. Because of their financial power, HMOs are able to negotiate favourable deals with providers on behalf of their subscribers. But as already noted, HMOs go further than a bit of tough bargaining with physicians and hospitals to get a percentage shaved off the price of a consultation or operation. Through a system of budget setting, bonus payments, withholds and referral funds, HMOs have tied health-care providers into a fairly strict financial regime.

There are many different types of HMO, employing different financial controls and structured in different ways in terms of their organization and management. Although beginning their life as Pre-Paid Group Practices largely set up by US workers along the lines of European sick-fund organizations, over the last 20 years the managed health-care movement has developed and adapted. There are now four basic managed health-care systems operating in the USA: the staff, group, individual practice association (IPA) and network models. As Weiner and Ferris and others have noted, it is difficult to draw a unified picture of the financial arrangements between managed health-care organizations/arrangements due to the sheer variety of managed health-care plans on offer. A brief look at the typical financial arrangements within the four basic types of HMOs provides a reasonably comprehensive picture however.

Staff model HMOs

In staff model HMOs, physicians tend to be salaried, and work to a specific contract laying down work practices, etc. Staff model HMOs usually provide care at one large, clinic-like base. Doctors often participate in profit-sharing arrangements as well. With doctors on fixed salaries (fixed in terms of an inability of doctors to radically alter their income solely through their own, clinical, actions) the financial incentives are very different from traditional fee-per-item of service. As employees of the HMO, doctors have more of an incentive to control the financial consequences of their clinical decisions because their salaries depend on the financial viability of the HMO as a whole. On top of this, profit-sharing further encourages doctors to treat patients efficiently, avoiding unnecessary referrals to secondary care, etc.

Group model HMOs

In group model HMOs, doctors form a group independent of the HMO. The HMO acts as the financial intermediary between the patient/subscriber and the health-care provider. The HMO sets up contracts with physicians – who only contract with a single HMO. One of the largest HMOs in the USA – Kaiser Permanente – is a typical example of a group model-managed care organization. Kaiser is the legally distinct, HMO corporation, and Permanente is the multispecialty group practice. As with other sorts of HMOs, the group model sets up contracts with physicians. The HMO creates budgets to fund different forms of care (e.g. primary, secondary, pharmacy, etc) based on actuarial formulae which use factors such as age, sex and sometimes previous patterns of health-care resource utilization by HMO subscribers. The primary care physicians contracted to the HMO act as gatekeepers to other forms of care, and work within the monthly capitated budgets set by the HMO.

Over- and under-spending by primary care physicians are dealt with by using a 'withhold' fund. In a sense this fund represents the shared financial risk between the doctor and the HMO. If, at the end of the year, a physician is under-spent, then the physician's withhold fund is paid back to the physician. In addition, the physician may receive a bonus payment if the HMO as a whole is in surplus. On the other hand, an over-spent physician may only receive part of their withhold (the rest being used to offset the over-spending) and no bonus payment. If a physician or practice continually over-spends the HMO may terminate their contract.

IPA HMOs

Individual practice association (IPA) HMOs originally consisted of usually single-handed practices, traditionally carrying out fee-per-item of service work, who wished to compete with the emerging staff/group HMOs. IPAs devised their own pre-paid plans (similar to other forms of HMOs). The key to the emergence of IPAs was the competition from other forms of HMOs, and not the desire to contain costs *per se*. Many IPAs also continue to supply fee-per-item of service work to their patients.

Network model HMO

The network model HMO is really just an extension of the IPA model, moving closer to the group practice form of HMO. IPA/network model HMOs are groupings of distinct practices able to offer a greater range of services to patients and contracting with more than one HMO. Many of the financial arrangements used by group practice HMOs are also used by IPA/network HMOs.

Organization of HMOs

The variety of financing methods which exist within the HMO/ managed care movement is reflected in the organizational structure of HMOs. HMOs can exist as non-profit-making corporations right up to organizations which are essentially run by mother hospitals (with the obvious links in terms of HMO subscribers being referred to the parent hospital). Around one-third of all HMOs are non-profit organizations, but, as Weiner and Ferris point out, this one-third accounts for over 50 per cent of all HMO subscribers. Some HMOs are owned by insurance companies, others by consumers themselves or groups of doctors.

Given the large employer contribution to the US's medical insurance bill, many big firms have set up their own managed health-care plans based on the HMO model. As with much of the US health-care industry, to UK eyes the sheer plurality of systems is staggering, and is summed up by Weiner and Ferris:

> . . . the US HMO Industry is made up of some strange bedfellows. At one end of the spectrum are single-site, non-profit consumer-oriented collectives that initially saw themselves as socialised alternatives to the insurance company/ AMA dominated big business of private practice. At the other end are multi-site chains that are subsidiaries of multi-billion dollar for-profit corporations.

This is not so much an ABC health-care economy as an ABCDEFG . . . XYZ economy.

HOW HAS THE MANAGED HEALTH-CARE MOVEMENT MANAGED?

In one sense, the HMO movement has managed extremely well. Judged by the number of HMOs and HMO-type organizations (over 1500 managed health-care plans are currently in existence in the USA) and the number of people now enrolled in one form of managed health-care organization or another (50–55 per cent of all Americans), the managed health-care movement has become the dominant health-care system in the USA.

For HMOs, growth has been dramatic: in 1985, there were around 400 HMOs with some 19 million subscribers. In the following two years, the number of HMOs rose from 600 to about 650, and subscribers increased from 24 million to 28 million. HMOs have also undergone some structural change since the beginning of the 1980s. In 1980, for instance, of the 5 per cent of the US population enrolled with HMOs, around 20 per cent were enrolled with IPA HMOs, and the remaining 80 per cent with staff/group HMOs. By 1989, however, the IPA/network HMO had become the dominant form of HMO, accounting for 60 per cent of subscribers, compared with 40 per cent in staff/group HMOs.

Part of the reason for the current dominance of HMOs can be attributed to the spur they received from federal and state subsidies in the early 1980s in an attempt to find some form of financing system which was less prone to the medical cost inflation that had been draining state and federally-funded Medicare and Medicaid programmes. Similar reasons prompted the private insurance market to push for reorganization of health-care financing. State subsidies also partly explain the shift in the popularity of staff/group HMOs to IPA/network HMOs. Subsidies in the early 1980s were primarily channelled into non-profit HMOs who were forced, by and large, into hiring their own doctors because of the boycott of HMOs by many private physicians. Thus, staff/group HMOs predominated at first. However, for some years now subsidies have been withdrawn, and given the comparatively high cost of setting up an HMO from scratch, it is easier and cheaper to set up an IPA/network HMO based on existing practices.

Although there were other reasons for the growth in HMOs, such as consumer preference for the types of services HMOs offered etc., the fundamental impetus for growth came from an increasingly pressing need to contain costs. If cost containment was the driving force behind the HMO and managed health-care movement, then what has happened to health-care costs over the last 20 years or so and have there been any costs associated with this particular approach to containment? Specifically, what changes have there been in terms of the type, level and, importantly, distribution of health-care services?

Cost containment: limited success?

One of the difficulties of identifying the effects of HMOs, and the managed health-care movement in general, on costs is that many changes have been happening simultaneously in the US health-care system. Chapter 5 listed a few of the regulatory mechanisms introduced by the state over the last 20 years as well as changes in the private insurance market. Disentangling the effects of all these changes is not easy. Furthermore, as Robinson (1990) says in reporting Fuchs (1988), it may be too early to say whether cost-containment policies (including HMOs) have been successful or not, or whether any effects they do have will be long lasting.

There have been literally hundreds of studies examining the effects of the changing health-care market structure, regulation, etc. on costs over the last ten years. But before reviewing some of this evidence, in order to be clear what cost containment means, it is perhaps worth reiterating Pauly's (1988) argument that competition (and this includes HMOs) may not automatically lead to cost containment in global terms. Pauly has argued that competition may minimize costs given some specific level and quality of health care provided, but consumer preference may be such that higher quality and/or levels of service are demanded, hence pushing up costs and expenditure. Pauly is restating a truism about markets and the interaction of demand and supply: at the *micro* level competition may reduce costs, but at the *macro* level total costs (or rather, expenditure) will be a combination of demands placed on suppliers by consumers, and suppliers' ability/willingness to meet those demands. This is the essence of the privatization of the decision 'how much should be spent on health care?'

Given Pauly's reminder of one of the basic characteristics of the market, examining the global trends in US health-care expenditure for evidence of the effects of cost-containment policies such as HMOs would be inappropriate. A number of studies have looked at costs at the micro level, however, and some of these are reviewed below.

Weiner and Ferris report conclusions from Luft (1981) and Manning *et al.* (1984) that HMOs do appear to be cost effective systems, with cost savings averaging 5–30 per cent compared with traditional fee-per-item of service practice. As Weiner and Ferris point out, of course, given that many of the services under fee-per-item of service are provided at higher costs than in the UK, it is not clear that HMO-type systems in the UK would have such significant (if any) effects on costs in the NHS.

Although there is evidence that HMOs have exerted a downward pressure on costs, this evidence is by no means consistent. For example, Hilman (1987) and Moore (1979) have examined the financial incentives faced by physicians working in or with HMOs. They suggest that these stick/carrot incentives do not always work in the way the HMO intended. One example which has been well identified in the literature about cost containment is 'DRG creep'. In the USA, DRGs (diagnosis related groups) have been a popular method of categorizing patients on admission and have been adapted to fit in with the predetermined price schedules used by HMOs as a basis for reimbursing hospitals. They are also widely used for reimbursement under Medicare's prospective payment system (PPS). Essentially, DRGs classify patients into one of around 500 categories set up in such a way that the costs of treating patients in any one category will be more or less the same. So, different DRGs imply different levels of resource use. The incentive structure is clear: patients admitted to hospital in essence carry with them a fixed budget and it is in the hospital's interest to provide care in such a way that these individual budgets are not exceeded. However, the system depends on the accurate assigning of patients to DRGs on admission. It is here that 'DRG creep' enters. There is a significant temptation to 'over-categorize' patients, that is, assign them to a slightly more expensive DRG than may be strictly necessary in terms of the treatment they are likely to need. There is yet another parallel here with the reforms of the NHS where there is a potential temptation in some cases for hospitals to classify extra-contractual referral (ECR) patients (i.e. those whose district of residence do not hold contracts with the admitting hospital) as emergency cases – which, under the new system, must be paid for by the district of residence.

The counter to DRG creep and other methods of circumventing HMOs' financial controls, has been the introduction and/or tightening of utilization reviews, pre-admission approvals, etc. To a certain extent these policies overcome abuse of the system, but, as Long and Welch (1988) point out, health-care spending is a bit like a balloon – squeeze it in one place (e.g. hospital in-patients through the use of DRG prospective payments, URs, pre-admission approval, etc.) and it tends to bulge out somewhere else (where there is less price restriction, e.g. out-patient/ambulatory care).

Merril and McLaughlin (1986) examined the effects of competition in the health-care industry by looking at the extent of HMO penetration in a number of urban areas over the decade 1971 to 1981. Their results showed that areas of high competition – in terms of the concentration of HMOs – did not have lower costs. However, in relation to a specific, but significant health-care cost – physicians' incomes – Green (1988) notes that median net incomes fell by 5 per cent over the period 1975 to 1985. Green attributes this to the pressure placed on this cost by HMOs and other forms of managed care. For example, Green implies that as HMOs have become more numerous, so the opportunities for newly-qualified physicians to set up their own fee-per-item of service solo practices has become increasingly restricted.

In contrast to Merril and McLaughlin's study, Zwanziger and Melnick (1988) and Robinson and Luft (1988) have suggested that when looking at the period of greatest growth in HMOs (the 1980s), there is a discernible dampening of cost inflation. Both studies found that, compared with the 1970s, during the 1980s there was an increase in price competition as opposed to competition in terms of quality which in the past had tended to lead to increases in costs.

Robinson's conclusion (1990), was that as HMOs and other types of managed care organizations have learned the ropes of financial control, and as legislation (particularly a 1982 ruling allowing third-party payers – such as some forms of HMOs – to exclude providers from their participating lists) freed purchasers from certain constraints, so the cost-containment policies of the managed health-care system have begun to work.

Weiner and Ferris note, however, that there have recently been some setbacks to these policies, which have necessitated some change in direction on the part of the managed health-care movement. The financial risk-sharing between HMO and physician – which has been a central part of HMOs' financial control strategy – has run into some problems as it has increasingly been perceived that a potential trade off exists between financial control and quality/level of care.

Side effects of cost containment

The tension between controlling costs on the one hand, and meeting legitimate health-care needs in an appropriate and adequate manner on the other, certainly does not only exist in the managed health-care movement. It is a dilemma all health-care systems face. And all systems face a difficulty in trying to strike the right balance. In the USA, Weiner and Ferris report that there have been a number of million-dollar law suits which have specifically claimed that HMOs' financial incentives have led physicians to provide too few or inappropriate services, and in turn contributed to medical negligence.

There is some support for the views of litigants in these cases from a study by Ware *et al.* (1986). The study compared health outcomes of two groups of patients assigned to three different forms of health-care system: HMOs, a traditional fee-per-item of service where there was a degree of cost sharing (i.e. patients paid part of the cost of their care) and a fee-per-item of service system which offered free care at the time of use. On various measures of health outcome, the study found that 'non-poor' people fared well under HMOs; high-income people fared even better, but low-income people fared less well with the HMO compared with the free, fee-per-item of service. Ware *et al.* suggest that the poor may find themselves at a disadvantage (not helped perhaps by a degree of paternalism on the part of the medical profession) if they are not sophisticated users of health-care services.

As stated earlier, devising complex financial mechanisms, sharing financial risk and employing utilization reviews, etc. is one way of encouraging efficiency and hence reducing costs. Another way is, of course, to only admit patients to a health plan who are comparatively healthy and hence less costly to the HMO. There is evidence that this biased selection has occurred in the managed health-care movement. For example, it is only in recent years that HMOs have been signing up elderly people on any scale.

Managed health care and equity

This chapter started with the assertion that health care, or the efficient production of health care (or, for that matter, the efficient production of health) was not the only desirable outcomes from a health-care system; some notion of equity (equality of access, equality of outcome of treatment) was also important. Although there are some arguments to justify the equity assertion (these were noted in Chapter 5), by and large the assertion must remain an assertion which one either believes in or one does not.

For HMOs and the managed health-care system in general, equity has not, traditionally at least, been a particularly high priority. The system in which HMOs have developed has not been one in which equity – as anyone who has experienced the UK NHS – has played an underlying or key role. Moreover, it should be remembered that one of the main forces behind the creation of HMOs was the pressing need to contain costs. Given this background, it is perhaps not surprising that the managed health-care movement, despite its popularity, does not appear to have made any significant dent in the inequality of access to health-care facilities which is apparent from the large numbers of uninsured and inadequately insured Americans. But it is not just at the macro level that access inequality is still a significant issue. At the micro level of the individual HMO, a number of studies have shown that there is a degree of 'biased selection' of patients (e.g. Wilensky and Rossiter, 1986). Creaming off the better risks is a well-known way for insurers – any type of insurers – to limit their payouts. For HMOs, like any health-care insurance entity, selecting subscribers who are less likely to consume health care is one way of cutting costs. Given the trade off between the possibility of making a loss (and perhaps eventually going out of business) if they do not engage in biased patient selection, and reducing equality of access if they do, HMOs quite naturally will tend to choose the latter course.

Although there have been studies (e.g. Manning *et al.* 1984) which suggest that even after controlling for biased patient selection, patients are treated more efficiently by HMOs than by other forms of health care (such as traditional fee-per-item of service), for patients who have not been selected such knowledge is probably of little comfort. Furthermore, as is shown by the Ware *et al.* (1986) study, HMOs do not treat patients from lower social classes as well as those from higher social classes.

On balance, and despite some evidence that HMOs are perhaps better at delivering care to the poor than other non-HMO health-care organizations (Spitz and Abramson, 1987), for HMOs the business imperative tends to win out over any ethical imperative such as equity.

Clinton's reforms

The latest set of changes for the US health care system look likely to be one of the most radical shake-ups yet. The reform package – the Health Security Act – put together by Hillary Rodham Clinton with advice from a selected group of health policy analysts and political advisors was outlined in September 1993, and attempts to deal with the twin problems of poor coverage and access as well as escalating costs of health care.

One of the Act's main proposals is the imposition of compulsory health insurance coverage (to be paid by employers and employees) and extra government spending to extend coverage to the 37 million Americans currently under or uninsured. The Act – which has to negotiate a laborinthyne passage through the Senate and House of representatives – also plans to tackle the thorny issue of specifying a minimum package of care all Americans should be entitled to. The $350 billion the plan is estimated to cost over the next five years will be partly paid for by savings in current federal and state insurance schemes such as Medicaid and Medicare. In addition, extra taxes on cigarettes and alcohol are expected to further offset the plan's extra costs. The Act, in one form or another, is expected to come into force in 1997 – although the president has indicated that it will be important to get all parties – clinicians, insurance companies, employers and the public at large – to agree on the final shape of the reforms, and this could take time.

CONCLUSION

Perhaps one of the main observations to be made from this discussion of HMOs and their offspring is that they are rooted in, and originate from, a particular health-care system, which had its own unique history and development, and which had particular (if not wholly unique) problems to do with the financing of health care. The HMO experience illustrates that whilst market-based health-care systems seem able to change and adapt quickly (in the US case, to problems of escalating health-care costs), the results of this change are by no means perfect. This does not necessarily mean that further changes will not occur (they are certain to do so) or that these further changes will not represent improvements – measured as greater efficiency, improved access or whatever. It may be, as Fuchs (1988) has said, too early to pass judgement on the effects of the managed health-care movement.

Nevertheless, as Robinson (1990) has noted, as the cost-containment policies of state regulation and managed health care have begun to bite, the trade off between efficiency and equity/quality have been brought more sharply into focus. Furthermore, the ability of the US health-care market to adapt to the point where it can deal equitably with the millions of US citizens who, at the beginning of the 1990s, still remain uninsured or underinsured, is questionable.

7

MANAGING THE MARKET: THE WEST GERMAN EXPERIENCE

In Chapter 6, the US experience has been outlined. Meanwhile, back in Europe, health-care financing has grown and developed in a different way. Interestingly enough, there are links between one of the commonest forms of health-care system in Europe – social insurance – and the origins of health maintenance organizations (HMOs) in the USA. HMOs – which were originally called Pre-Paid Group Practices (PPGPs), but which underwent a name change for marketing purposes – started their lives as attempts by groups of US workers to copy the European sick funds they had known before emigration. But, if the rather heterogeneous US health-care 'system' – still in transition, still changing at a considerable pace – is at one end of the scale, then the West German National Health Insurance (NHI) system is perhaps at the other end, representing rock-like stability by comparison. In fact, it is probably the most stable system in the world. Since its invention in the early 1880s, the NHI has survived, virtually unscathed, a number of political, military, economic and social upheavals. It would seem that it must be doing something right. Over its lifetime (which is two-and-a-half times longer than the UK NHS) the NHI entitlement programme has increased the population it covers from around 10 per cent in 1883 to over 90 per cent in 1985 (Altensetter, 1986) and 'now provides fairly comprehensive coverage for all risks of chronic and temporary illness and physical, mental, or emotional disability as well as income-protection' (Altensetter, 1986). If the German system is doing something right (or at least, appears to have a life expectancy far greater than most other systems), then what is it? And why isn't everyone doing it? The answer to the latter question is that many countries are doing it, having imported (and suitably modified) Bismarck's original nineteenth-century health-care social insurance plans for their own use. In the European Community, only three countries do not have health-care systems based around some kind of social insurance or sick fund programme – Denmark, Ireland and the UK.

The answer to the former question, plus discussion of the issues raised by social insurance, takes up the rest of this chapter.

SOCIAL INSURANCE

Before looking in detail at the West German social insurance system, it is worth defining 'social insurance'. In fact, most social insurance systems – as in France, or The Netherlands, or Germany – have little or nothing to do with the actuarial concept of insurance at all. That is, the term 'insurance' is not so much a technical description of a system based on the assessments of risk, but is used in a more colloquial way to suggest 'protection'. Private health-care insurance (or for that matter, car insurance, house insurance, etc.) is based as closely as possible on individuals' actuarial risks. So, if you are old or suffer from a chronic medical condition which requires medical attention, then your private health-care premiums will be correspondingly higher than if you are young and fit. Such 'experience rating' is not used by most social insurance programmes. Instead, health care is usually financed through a specific tax on the incomes of those in work. Payment of this tax (it seems misleading to call it 'insurance') is usually compulsory. Medical benefits under social insurance are usually granted in kind, as opposed to the financial compensation for costs incurred more commonly provided by private insurance.

The key difference between social insurance systems and those based predominantly on a private insurance model hinges on differences in the underlying attitudes to access and equality, with all the overarching state regulation that these attitudes imply. In this respect, one may wonder what the differences are between social insurance and the UK NHS. Indeed, are there any differences? In financing terms, the difference is broadly that the NHS is financed from general taxation and not from a specific national insurance tax (the separate national insurance paid by employees and employers only contributes around 15 per cent of total NHS spending and is not, nor ever has been, specific to the NHS). There are then specific differences in the way doctors and hospitals are reimbursed for the care they provide. In France, for example, treatment costs are generally paid directly by patients, who then claim all or part of their expenses back from the state. Health care is generally not free at the point of use.

Social insurance in Germany

Although the German social insurance system is now over one hundred years old, its origins predate the creation of the German state. In 1849, legislation in Prussia set up statutory health-care insurance for workers in a number of industries. But it was under the first chancellor of Germany, Otto von Bismarck, that social insurance came to prominence. Legislation in 1883, 1884 and 1889, created a social insurance system covering various aspects of health, old age and unemployment for workers and their dependants.

Iglehart (1991) suggests that Bismarck had two reasons for instituting social insurance. The first was an attempt to quell social unrest amongst workers who were flocking to cities as a result of the industrial revolution. Bismarck's scheme was a way of buying political support from workers in exchange for the economic and social protection offered by social insurance. For most workers it was the former protection which was most valued, with health-care insurance considered as only secondary importance. The second reason was also political, but perhaps more 'moral', and underlay a greater range of the German state's activities than just social insurance. Iglehart quotes Rosenberg (1986) on this:

> The idea of this policy [social insurance] started by Bismarck was that the welfare of people does not result automatically out of economic growth in a free-market economy; the distribution has to be regulated, and the state should not limit itself to providing economic freedom.

There was thus a very early recognition that markets, whilst good at many things, are not, if left to their own devices, necessarily very good at everything, and in particular cannot be relied upon to promote the 'social solidarity' that Bismarck felt was needed for a politically stable, socially creditable and economically successful nation.

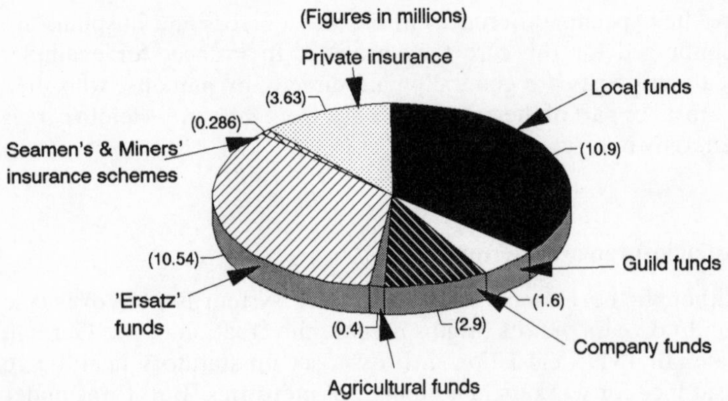

Figure 7.1 Membership (in millions) of private and social insurance schemes in Germany.
Source: Iglehart (1991).

Sickness funds and doctors' associations

Bismarck's original legislation created non-profit-making sickness funds whose job not only included the collection of national health insurance, but also the provision of health care. The employment of physicians by sickness funds was to give way, however, to the creation of panels of physicians who administered the payment of ambulatory care physicians (i.e. non-hospital doctors) on behalf of the sickness funds. These panels were later formally recognized as regional associations who now not only administer payments to physicians, but also negotiate fee schedules with the sickness funds.

In addition to the regional associations and the sickness funds, there is a second physicians' association representing hospital-based doctors – the Marburgerbund. There is a sharp distinction between the two physicians' associations both in terms of medical practice (ambulatory care physicians are not allowed to treat patients in hospital, for example) and in terms of the method of remuneration (see below).

Today, there are around 1200 sickness funds which, together with the regional associations, control the financial arrangements of the social insurance system which ensures that around 88 per cent of the

German population receive health care when needed. The remaining 12 per cent of the population insure themselves through the private medical insurance sector. Sickness funds are generally based on localities, 'substitute funds', occupations or companies (see Figure 7.1).

Source of finance

The main source of health-care financing (about 95 per cent) – essentially the income for sickness funds – comes from employers and employees in the form of a percentage of employees gross income (i.e. a pay-roll tax). Before 1950, employees paid two-thirds of their contribution to their sickness fund and employers one-third. Now, however, the burden is equally shared. Each fund sets its own contribution level for its own members. Typically, the combined contribution from employees and employers averages 13 per cent of an employee's gross wage. But this can vary, not only from year to year within the same fund, but also within the same year between funds. Iglehart quotes rates varying between 8 per cent and 16 per cent. There are a number of reasons for these variations. Funds need to set contribution rates at the beginning of the year to take account of two main factors: first, anticipated expenditure over the coming financial year, and secondly, the state of the labour market (in essence, the tax base). Health-care expenditure can vary between funds due to differences in the age structures of the different populations covered by funds or any of a multitude of social, economic or cultural factors which can affect the use of, or need for, health care. Because contributions are levied as a percentage of earnings, variations in rates can also occur due to disparities in average wage levels between different geographical areas. Differences in contribution rates are a sensitive political issue and are further discussed later.

Contribution to sickness funds is compulsory for everyone earning less than DM56 700 (about £21 000) a year. Those earning more can opt for private medical insurance or remain within a fund. However, many choose to remain with the sickness funds. Also, although there is a certain amount of switching between funds (perhaps to take advantage of differences in contribution rates), the vast majority of the population remain in the same fund all their lives.

The important difference between private medical insurance and social insurance is that the latter sets its 'premiums' on the basis of income, not health status. Germans who opt for private medical insurance (generally the affluent and civil servants who top up the care paid for them directly by the state) pay premiums based on actuarial risks. Interestingly, however, once signed up, the insured generally do not pay higher premiums as they get older, but stick with the premium level appropriate for their age when they started with the insurance. Premiums do rise, but only to reflect general rises in health-care costs. So, even in the private insurance market there is some redistribution of income in kind from the young/fit to the old/unfit.

Level of financing

Although international comparisons of health-care spending can be misleading because of differences in national accounting practices, problems with conversion to common comparative units etc., it does appear that spending per head in Germany is relatively high (see Table 4.2). It should be remembered that a proportion of NHI collected by sickness funds – about 7 per cent – is spent on cash benefits in order to offset lost income during illness. Whilst spending is high, there are those (generally the third-party payers) who think it unnecessarily high, and have acted to contain costs. This issue is discussed below.

Coverage

Although the great bulk of health-care financing comes from the NHI levied on employees and employers, the health-care system covers the whole population and not just those in work and contributing to the sickness funds. The funds cover the dependants of workers as well as others who do not work. In 1990, about 7 per cent of the workforce was unemployed. However, a combination of federal and local payments to sickness funds ensured that the unemployed (and their dependants) still received the same benefits as those in work. (In fact, equality of entitlement is guaranteed by law.)

Contributions for people who are retired are paid by pension funds in the form of a flat percentage rate equivalent to the national average contribution paid by those in employment. Because the elderly make disproportionately greater use of health-care services than other age groups, and certainly in excess of the national average, the pension funds' contribution invariably falls short of actual spending. In 1989, these contributions only covered 40 per cent of actual costs. The remaining 60 per cent is paid for by the sickness funds (essentially a redistribution from younger, fitter, employed people). Some funds with large numbers of retired people as members receive additional money from a national reserve to help keep down the general contribution rate.

Financing of ambulatory and hospital care

There are three separate methods by which health care is actually paid for. First, ambulatory care physicians (over half of whom are specialists rather than generalists) are reimbursed by their regional associations (acting on behalf of the sickness funds) in arrears, on a fee-per-item of service basis. These fees are based on a schedule previously negotiated between the regional association and the sickness funds.

Secondly, hospital-based physicians receive salaries, paid for out of money received by hospitals from sickness funds. Hospitals themselves are paid on the basis of a fixed per diem sum which varies according to the type of treatment provided. There is a fairly high degree of negotiation which has to take place between hospitals and sickness funds over these per diem costs and over other aspects of their budgets, however. Legislation enacted in 1985 introduced a prospective payment system for hospitals based on anticipated occupancy rates. Not only do hospitals negotiate with sickness funds over future occupancy rates (and hence the size of their budget), but also over the fee schedule for the per diem payments.

Finally, capital financing – money for buildings, large items of equipment, etc. – comes mainly from the state rather than from sickness funds. This is not only the case for state hospitals, but also the private sector (which constitutes about 4 per cent of all hospital beds). Both public- and private-sector capital works are subject to state-controlled planning.

SOCIAL INSURANCE: THE ANSWER?

It is evident that the German social insurance-based health-care system operates at some distance from the more market-oriented

US system, and in many respects (for instance, the underlying ethos of universal coverage) resembles more closely the UK NHS (there are also, of course, notable differences between the German application of social insurance and the NHS). It also appears that social insurance has been successful in securing high-quality health care for the entire German population (excluding the 9 per cent or so of earners who use private insurance) at an apparently socially acceptable level of financing. However, social insurance, at least the German variety, is not without its problems. These are discussed below.

The contributors

The main sources of health-care finance in Germany are employees and employers. Both share the burden of national health insurance equally (however, there are some cases where the employer must pay the whole contribution – for employees on low wages, for example). Currently, contributions average about 13 per cent of a worker's gross wage, but, as noted earlier, contributions vary between sickness funds (from around 8 to 16 per cent) for a variety of reasons. An important issue arising from this method of financing is the effect it has on the wider economy and its effects on the distribution of post-tax income.

In connection with the possible application of social insurance in the UK, Ludbrook and Maynard (1988) point out that in a competitive labour market, the conventional economic textbook analysis of the kind of split payment involved in national health insurance is that the burden of the tax/insurance eventually falls on the employee in terms of a reduced real wage. That is, employers tend to pass on their share of the payment of the insurance either to consumers (through price rises) and/or reduce the total cost of their payments by holding down wages (on which the insurance contributions are based). In the long run, it is argued, employees end up paying the entire amount of the insurance through a combination of direct payments (i.e. the actual deduction of their share of the insurance from their wages) and indirect payments (i.e. a further combination of lower wages and higher prices). In fact, it is not just the employed who bear the burden of higher prices. Those on fixed incomes, the retired and others on state benefits will also contribute to the sickness funds indirectly through higher prices.

The simple 50:50 split between employer and employee is

therefore not as straightforward as it first appears. Whether or not it matters that in the long run employees (and others not in work, but consuming goods and services) end up paying the bulk of NHI depends on views/policies about such things as the equality of distribution of income and wider economic goals such as international competitiveness.

Another issue which concerns contributions is related to the disparities in rates set by different sickness funds. For local funds covering fixed geographical areas, there can be marked differences in the level of contributions arising from differences in the labour market. Those in employment in areas with below-average earnings are likely to have to contribute proportionally more to their sickness funds than workers in areas with above-average earnings. Similarly, areas with above-average populations of elderly retired people need to set rates which are higher than areas with below-average numbers of elderly. Although there is a national reserve which recompenses funds with disproportionate numbers of elderly members, this does not necessarily leave all funds on an equal footing and there is currently a fairly charged debate in Germany over the resolution of the different 'risk structures' different sickness funds face in terms of age, sex, tax base, etc. And it is likely that the debate will eventually lead to some reforms in the NHI system (Hencke, 1990).

Cost containment

Despite its remarkable stability, the German health-care system has not been immune from cost inflation. Since the late 1970s, central government has passed a number of measures aimed at controlling health-care costs in an essentially open-ended system. With no cash limits and with high patient expectations of health-care services, (there have been perennial problems for sickness funds in raising enough income to cover actual costs.) Altensetter (1986) notes that even after the payment of subsidies to hospitals to make up the difference between sickness funds' incomes and the actual costs of treating patients coming through the NHI scheme, hospitals were still not fully recompensed for their services. (The reason for this was that subsidies were calculated on notional estimates of what costs a particular hospital *should* incur rather than the costs they *actually* incurred. This is similar in many ways to the calculation of central government grant to local authorities in the UK. Ultimately, as

Altensetter points out, the not-inconsiderable responsibility for ensuring that hospitals (both public and private) received enough to cover their costs fell to those mandated agents responsible for providing their local populations with adequate health-care services – the local municipalities and counties.

Although Germans have always had to make some contribution towards the cost of certain prescriptions, dental treatment, etc. (as in the UK), in recent years these payments have been raised in an attempt to contain costs overall. Currently, these contributions represent about 7.5 per cent of total revenue collected by sickness funds. Other cost-containment measures – which reflect some of the measures taken in the USA – include greater scrutiny of physicians' medical practices by third-party payers such as the sickness funds, private insurers, etc. There have also been recent moves to try and restrict what is believed to be a certain amount of overconsumption (i.e. unnecessary treatment) on the part of the German population. Compared with many other European countries, Germans appear to have quite a high propensity to consume health care. Hospitalization rates and mean length of stay in hospital tend to be high compared with other countries, and utilization of physician services as measured by the number of contacts per person per year is twice as high as in the UK (see Figure 7.2). Although there are a number of reasons for this (and indeed, high admission and utilization rates and lengths of stay could be seen as good for patients rather than bad for the system), there is undoubtedly an incentive on the part of ambulatory care physicians and hospitals to 'over-prescribe' arising from the way these groups are reimbursed for their services.

As will be recalled, physicians are generally paid on a fee per item of service basis by sickness funds (via the regional associations). As has been well documented in other countries with similar reimbursement systems (Canada, USA, etc.), physicians invariably take the opportunity to control their incomes offered by fee per item of service by increasing their service (and hence their incomes). In fact, German doctors' incomes have been amongst the highest in the world. For example, in 1980, out of 11 major OECD countries, their earnings as a multiple of GDP per person (at 7.5) ranked higher than their US and Canadian counterparts, and over twice the level of most other countries, including the UK (Parkin, 1989). However, since 1980 doctors' earnings have been falling, and now stand at around 3.5 times average GDP per head. This fall in income relative to the population as a whole is due partly to a rise in

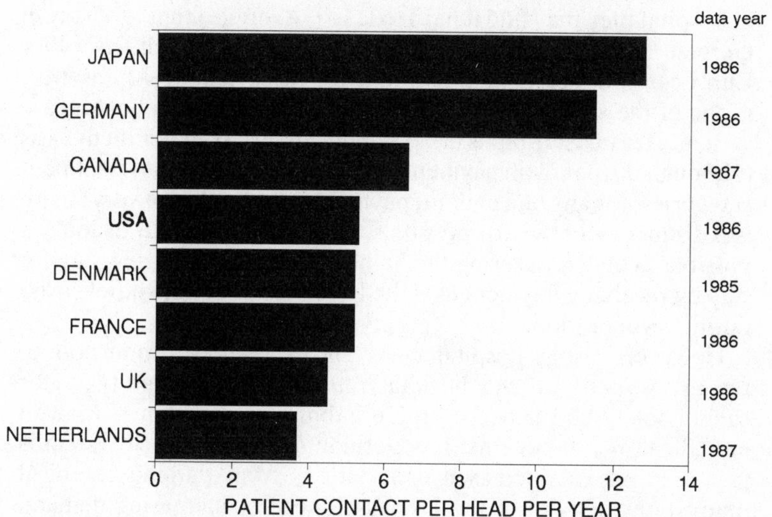

Figure 7.2 Patient contact: consultations and visits per head for selected countries.

Source: Sondier (1990).

the number of physicians (during a time of little population growth), limiting perhaps the scope for doctors to increase their incomes, and partly due to the recognition by, and action of, third-party payers who pushed for closer scrutiny of physicians' medical practices as well as a voucher scheme for patients placing certain restrictions on hospital referrals (although this latter measure has not been very successful).

Culyer (1976), has conjectured that the system of remuneration for community physicians may have also contributed to the comparative lack of out-patient services in Germany and the much greater specialization of community physicians than elsewhere in Europe. In turn, the lack of out-patient facilities may have also contributed to the high rates of hospital admission compared with the rest of Europe. In addition, the remunerative system may also discourage the use of (generally cheaper) preventative treatments.

But if German patients perhaps find it hard to escape their community physicians' surgeries without having undergone a fistful of tests and treatment that was not perhaps strictly necessary, once in hospital they may find it hard to leave. Average lengths of stay in German hospitals are considerably higher than in many other European countries, and their reduction, according to Altensetter, is one of the keys to cost containment for the German health-care system. Because hospitals are reimbursed on a fixed per diem basis (although the per diem payments vary according to broad treatment categories, for any one patient, payments per day do not vary) there is a distinct incentive for hospitals to retain patients for as long as possible, hence recovering the higher costs of the first few days of stay by receiving payments for the lower costs (mainly hotel costs) during recuperation.

However, rising hospital costs and a greater proportion of resources spent on the hospital rather than community sector cannot solely be blamed on the reimbursement systems. As with most health-care systems, the German social insurance system is just as prone to increased expectations from patients, medical innovations and, as in the UK as elsewhere, increasing demand from growing numbers of elderly people. But to these can be added the comparative lack of control over spending by sickness funds; the strong influence of the medical profession over the level of spending, what it is spent on and for whom; and an underlying ethos of provision of whatever service regardless of cost.

Finally, it should be remembered that cost containment, in itself, is not a particularly sensible policy, eventually leading to the absurd conclusion that nothing at all should be spent. The real issue or question for the German health-care system, as for other countries' systems, is whether there is *unnecessary* spending. That is, it is a question of opportunity cost; money spent on unnecessary care and treatment is money not spent on *necessary* care and treatment. It is in this sense of the meaning of cost containment that the Germans are tackling rising levels of spending. Whilst the social insurance system has no ready or automatic answers to the difficult macro decisions involved in determining appropriate levels of spending on health care compared with other desirable ways of committing scarce resources, or, within health care, the micro decisions and choices between different forms of care and treatment, the system itself does seem to allow a degree of discussion and debate about these matters. Having said that, social insurance, its supporting bureaucracy and its seemingly entrenched power bases (primarily the medical profession) do not lend themselves to change very easily. This is perhaps one reason for the system's stability.

Equity

As was noted in Chapter 5, there are a number of definitions of equity and a great number of ways of measuring it, especially concerning the delivery and/or consumption of health care. In terms of the financing of health care, there are two aspects of equity – vertical and horizontal. Vertical equity refers to the requirement that unequals (defined, perhaps, as the ability to pay) are treated unequally (in terms of their contribution to the financing of health care). But, as Wagstaff *et al.* (1989) note, although vertical equity tends to receive most attention in the economics literature, horizontal equity – that equals be treated equally – is also important.

So how does the German system fare in terms of the equity of its financing? The first point to note is that NHI payments (accounting for the vast bulk of expenditure on health care) are not related to health status; payments are not 'experience' related, but vary according to the level of a worker's income. High earners pay more than low earners in NHI as contributions are based on a percentage of earnings. For those in work and paying NHI, the contribution system is *proportional*; it is not *progressive* (the well-off pay proportionately more than the less well-off), nor is it *regressive* (the well-off pay proportionately less than the less well-off). Although not progressive, there is some redistribution from the rich to the poor in terms of the financing system. There is also some redistribution from earners to non-earners (e.g. the retired, the unemployed, etc.) which is likely to tip what is essentially a proportional system of financing into one which is progressive. However, because there is an upper earnings limit on compulsory contributions (currently set at around £21 000 p.a.), redistribution is, in theory at least, somewhat limited. Countering this, however, is the fact that most Germans earning over £21 000 tend to stay with their sickness funds rather than opting out completely from the NHI system.

The contribution system is complicated by the fact that different sickness funds levy different contribution rates. This can mean that neighbours earning exactly the same income but belonging to different sickness funds (one to an occupational group, and one to a local fund, for example) can end up paying different contributions.

Overall, therefore, it is not easy to judge the degree of equity in financing, but it is likely that there is a degree of inequity favouring the less wealthy. In terms of vertical equity, it is likely that unequals are treated unequally, with the less well-off paying less than the well-off. As Hencke (1990) admits, the exact degree of vertical inequity is difficult to assess, and has not been well quantified. However, contrary to this qualitative assertion, work by Wagstaff *et al.* suggests that for the social insurance component of the Dutch health-care system there is inequity favouring the rich. But contrary to this they found that the compulsory social insurance contributions for catastrophic illness – AWBZ premiums, another component of the overall social insurance system – were also inequitable, but this time favouring the less well-off.

In terms of horizontal equity, the example of the two neighbours suggests that theoretically at least, there is the possibility that equals (in terms of ability to pay) are not necessarily treated equally (in terms of contributions). The extent to which this is a significant occurrence is difficult to judge without a detailed analysis of incomes matched against contributions. However, given the two-fold variation in contribution rates across sickness funds it would seem likely that there is a degree of horizontal inequity in financing and that it may well not be insignificant.

As far as equity of the delivery and provision of health care is concerned, what evidence there is suggests that Germans enjoy a high degree of equality in terms of access and treatment. The unemployed, the retired and the families and dependants of those in work all have access to the same level of ambulatory and hospital care as those who work and who contribute directly to the NHI. Indeed, federal laws have been enacted to ensure that the unemployed and their dependants receive the same care as those in work. What inequalities do exist are likely to be more to do with factors unrelated to the financing system; the German middle class are unlikely to be much different from the UK middle class (or the US middle class) in making a more than proportionate use of health-care services than other groups, for example.

As with the UK's health-care system, the German system runs alongside a private health-care sector. However, apart from a suggestion that private patients (with private medical insurance) receive more prompt appointments (physicians and hospitals receive higher payments for private patients), there is not much to choose between the medical care provided to private and sickness fund patients. As in the UK, whilst there is the freedom to 'go private' there is a tendency, even amongst those who can afford to do so, to stick with the state system. Nevertheless, what the

Germans have (as do the British) is a two-tier health-care system, where the only conceivable reason for going private is that it offers benefits (not necessarily medical) over and above that offered by the state. Of course, the trade off here is between the freedom of individuals to spend their own money on the goods and services of their own choice, and the outlawing of the private health-care sector. Pragmatism wins out in both countries, but the cost is access for the rich to (possibly) better private care which is denied to the less well-off.

Equality of access and equality of treatment are perhaps not surprising given the placatory origins of the German social insurance system and the strong consensus which still survives amongst the key actors in the health-care system that equality is an important objective within the health-care field, not just with regard to health *per se*, but also for its contribution to social cohesion and social solidarity which underlie many other aspects of German life.

CONCLUSION

If there is one thing to be learned from the German health-care system it is that it is the *German* health-care system. Classifying health-care systems is notoriously difficult, and can easily lead to as many classifications as there are systems. The German system is based on a concept of social insurance, characterized by a highly decentralized approach to financing and an overarching regulatory system, and underpinned by a commitment to consensus, a powerful medical profession and a strong economy. Whilst individuals' annual payments to the NHI are 'transparent' (they can be identified separately on wage slips unlike spending on the NHS), cost-consciousness is not high amongst patients and physicians because the costs associated with individual treatments are dealt with in an opaque way by the reimbursement system.

There is no doubt that the German system has been successful. Health-care consumption is high, access appears fairly equitable, the problem of cost containment is not of the same order as in some other countries and the health of the population is generally good. The extent to which the particular organization of financing health care in Germany is responsible for this is debatable, however. How the system is structured, the organization of health-care providers, the attitudes of both providers and patients to health and health care, and the state of the economy at large are just some of the factors which influence the way the health-care system operates and help determine its success or failure (however measured). For example, whilst the wealth of a country is not always a good indicator of the equity of its health-care system (e.g. the USA), it is always easier (less painful) to redistribute when there is more, rather than less, to redistribute.

Whilst for Americans concerned about the state of the US health-care system, social insurance, German-style, appears to be an attractive alternative which does not stray too far from many aspects of the US set up, but at the same time seems to produce more desirable outcomes in terms of cost containment, equality of access, etc., from a UK perspective, the alternative is perhaps not so clear cut. It is not apparent, for example, that the German health-care system is any better than the UK NHS at addressing some of the fundamental problems of efficiency and equity which confront all health-care systems. Moreover, it is not always precisely clear (as this chapter has perhaps shown) exactly what makes one health-care system operate in the way it does or produce the effects it does (from the efficiency with which it produces health-care services to the degree of equality with which it distributes the results of its production). Even if all the multifarious factors can be identified, measured, and their exact contribution and interaction quantified, as Ludbrook and Maynard (1988) have shown, transition to a social insurance system (based on a pay-roll tax) in the UK is likely to come with considerable costs – regressive redistribution of post-tax income, reduction in aggregate demand in the economy, fall in the demand for labour and, possibly, a rise in prices. Not only are these likely to outweigh any potential benefits, it is not at all evident that a change of funding from tax to social insurance would either address one of the perceived main problems of the NHS (underfunding/low level of service activity) or produce any significant improvements in other areas (such as equality of access).

8

SOME VIEWS OF THE FUTURE

Although providing some general insights into the way health care can be financed, the foregoing reviews strongly indicate the often unique circumstances in which health-care systems have arisen and continue to operate. What this seems to suggest is that 'borrowing' health-care systems from one country to try and solve particular or perceived problems in another is likely to create just as many new problems as it solves (if indeed it even solves the perceived problems in the first place). Health care in the UK is currently undergoing some radical change in the way it is structured and in the way it is financed. Whilst there is some dispute as to the reasons (and indeed the need) for these changes, the origin of many of the reforms lies in ideas and practices underlying other health-care systems, although adapted to suit the particular environment in which the NHS has operated.

The first year of the NHS reforms was largely characterized by stability, with the NHS striving to emulate its previous patterns of service provision, patient flows, etc., despite the change in its economic environment. Nevertheless, the intention of the reforms is to change things. So how is the NHS likely to develop over the coming years? And in particular, how is the issue and practicalities of health-care financing likely to change given the new direction health care in the UK is now taking since the introduction of the NHS reforms?

This chapter will attempt to indicate a possible course towards the end of the century. There are many unknowns and (judging from past experience) many unpredictable events. However, as Chapter 2 showed, the current reforms of the NHS contain many seeds of change which suggest that health care in the UK could look very different by the year 2000.

Cock-up or conspiracy?

It is important to formulate some view of the origins of the NHS reforms, as an understanding of the history of the changes on which the NHS is now embarked can provide pointers to the potential outcome of these changes.

Along with the two views of what the NHS reforms would be ('not much change' and 'radical shake up' (see, for example, Chapter 1)), there are also two views or theories concerning the reasons for the reforms in the first place – conspiracy and cock-up (Timmins, 1988). But as with the former pair of theories, this latter pair probably overstate the real situation. The conspiracy view – that the NHS was deliberately starved of funds in the few years leading up to Margaret Thatcher's announcement of a review of the NHS in 1988 – suggests a degree of plotting and planning which is hard to believe. On the other hand, the cock-up theory – that the financial crisis of the winter of 1987 was in essence the result of a blunder by the Department of Health, compounded by a failure on the part of Health Ministers to go back to the Treasury for extra money and which led inevitably to the then Prime Minister's announcement – seems too random and too out of character with much else of Government policy towards the public sector at the time. For cock-up theorists, there is some evidence to suggest that the Government's NHS review was a result of a combination of external events which left them slightly wrong-footed. The Conservative Party manifesto for the June 1987 election made no mention of any review or shake-up of the NHS, for example. And there is something to be said for the genuine nature of the surprise that Ministers expressed as beds began to close and operations were cancelled at an alarming rate in the winter of 1987.

However, rather than history as blunder, confusion and mistake – favoured by Timmins in his review of his own newspaper articles during the NHS debate over 1987 and 1988 – or history as well-thought out, well-executed plans (usually favoured by the victors, and hence the history writers), what is favoured here is a mixture of the two extremes.

Chapter 1 referred briefly to an unpublished review of alternative sources of finance for the NHS. This review was conducted by senior civil servants from the Department of Health, the Treasury and other departments and carried out in 1981 at the behest of Health Ministers. The fact that such a review was carried out is not surprising; all governments carry out exercises designed to look at various policy options. Indeed, it would be somewhat worrying if they did not. However, whilst attaching too much importance to this initial 1981 review is perhaps dangerous (too conspiratorial), it seems clear that the view that the NHS was considered somehow politically unassailable and that the Government accidentally painted themselves into a corner over NHS financing from which the only escape was to announce a review of the NHS, is at least partially contradicted by the 1981 review. The Government at the time *were* considering alternative policies for financing the NHS and they had fairly clear ideas about the sorts of policy objectives they were aiming for. These included: promotion of the private health-care sector; tax concessions on health-care investment and private insurance; contracting out of state insurance; new and higher charges for NHS services; discontinuing parts of the NHS. In addition, the review was called on to investigate possibilities for changing the way health care was financed in the UK – including alternatives such as private insurance and a form of social insurance.

Whilst not wishing in any way to suggest that this early review represents the key, and unchanged, agenda with regard to the recent NHS reforms, it does at least indicate the beginning of a line of Governmental thinking which started much earlier than the eventual NHS reforms, and which paralleled other lines of thought and action with respect to the public sector as a whole at the time, and which, indeed, finally saw some of its investigations become reality with the passing of the 1990 NHS Act.

Mainly for the candid way in which it expressed its terms of reference, the 1981 review provides a useful starting point in looking at the future of health-care financing in the UK up to the turn of the century. The financial future of health care in the UK is examined under two main headings: sources of finance and levels of finance, and expands on issues raised in Chapter 2 which identified a number of policy changes contained in the NHS reforms which may perhaps develop in some unexpected ways.

SOURCES OF FINANCING

For over 40 years, the National Health Service has largely been financed from general taxation. In its first two years of existence all

NHS spending came from income tax. The 1950s saw some changes; patients started to be charged for certain services (prescriptions, dental treatment, etc.), national insurance contributions started to provide around 10 per cent of total spending, and local authorities financed and provided services through a combination of rates and central government grant. During the 1960s, the share of financing from taxation reached its lowest point, contributing around 70 per cent of total NHS spending. This low was matched by increased financing from NHS contributions (16 per cent) and payments by users of the NHS (5 per cent). In the 1970s services were transferred from local authorities to the NHS, and there was an adjusting rise in financing from taxation. But during this time the contribution to NHS finances from National Insurance fell to its lowest level (6 per cent), as did the contribution from patient charges (2 per cent). At the beginning of the 1980s the proportion of NHS spending financed from general taxation was nearly 89 per cent. By the end of the decade this had fallen to just over 77 per cent, and the contribution from National Insurance had returned to nearly 15 per cent. Income from patient charges remained almost static for most of the 1980s. Estimates for 1990–91 (DoH, 1991) suggested that patients would contribute nearly 6.5 per cent of the NHS revenue budget in the form of charges, however. The 1980s also saw the beginning of a trend in revenue raised through income generation schemes and asset sales (surplus land and buildings). By the end of the decade, the latter was contributing over one-third of total capital spending in the NHS.

So what of the 1990s? How are the six current main sources of funding of health care in the UK (taxation, national insurance, patient charges, income generation, private medical insurance and direct payments) going to change over the coming years? Are there any detectable or discernible trends in past patterns of financing? The answer to this last question is that there are, but they must be read in conjunction with other external factors shaping health-care financing policy. Bearing in mind that the future tends to look very similar to the present, and quite similar to the past, one conclusion that may be drawn from these trends in financing is that taxation has, and is likely to remain, the main source of funding for the NHS for the foreseeable future. This is not just based on the fact that taxation has in the past always been the main source of funding, but also on the reasons it has remained the main source of funding in the past.

Given the political decision to provide and run a state health-care service, funding that service from general taxation is not only comparatively cheap in administrative terms, but it draws on a wide and generally stable base, provides political flexibility in determining funding levels and is generally seen as an equitable way of raising finance in the first place. Moreover, changing to another form of financing may not only be more costly to administer in the long run, but carries transitional costs as well (cf. Ludbrook and Maynard's work on the costs of switching to social insurance, 1988). However, the crucial point here is what 'the decision to provide and run a state health-care service' actually means. What it does not necessarily mean is that all health care will be exclusively funded and provided by the state. And this is clear from the NHS reforms. The separation of purchasing from providing and the responsibility of District Health Authorities to ensure that their resident populations have access to a reasonable level of quality health-care services, does not mean that DHAs purchase exclusively from NHS providers. Equally, for NHS providers, the separation does not mean that they provide exclusively to NHS purchasers (DHAs and GP fundholders). But while general taxation is likely to remain the single most important source of funding health care in the UK, given the increased potential for other sources of financing as a result of the reforms of the NHS, as a proportion of total health-care funding general taxation is likely to fall over the next ten years.

Increased role for private financing

One particular source of health-care financing which has significant prospects for growth in the future is private funding, either through direct payments by individuals for health-care services or, as is more likely, via private medical insurance. Some industry analysts (HSJ, 1990, for example) have predicted that the number of insured individuals will rise from 13 per cent of the population at present, to over 50 per cent by the end of the century. Others are more sceptical, but still the consensus appears to be a continuation in previous growth trends.

There are many factors which, separately and together, influence the size of the private insurance sector and its prospects for expansion. For example, the perception of alternative sources of health care (i.e. the NHS), the affordability of premiums, the coverage of insurance policies, etc. In an investigation into private health care in the UK, Higgins (1988) reviewed the reported reasons why some people 'go private'. Although this question appertained to private treatment, it also applies to medical insurance which, when it is called upon, may now fund treatment in the private or public sector. Whilst Higgins found that very few studies actually asked patients why they went private, a survey by Horne (1984) of 307 private patients suggested that the primary motivation for going private was the avoidance of NHS waiting lists. Other factors such as choice of doctor, better nursing care, pre-arranged admission and additional services were mentioned much less frequently. However, the data in this area are somewhat confusing. The Chief Executive of the British United Provident Association (BUPA) in evidence to a House of Commons Expenditure Committee in 1971 (House of Commons, 1972) revealed that his own Association's research suggested that the abilities to fix a pre-arranged date for admission and choose a doctor were more important to private patients than jumping queues. Whilst there is disagreement over the specific reasons some people choose to go private, it is clear the general reason is that traditionally, private health care offers more, or is at least perceived to offer more, than the NHS. But will this always be the case?

NHS Trusts – looking for new sources of revenue?

One of the key actors on the provider side will be the NHS Trust. Whilst the first year of the reforms was heavily proscribed in terms of the degree of change the Department of Health was willing to allow (and, it should be added, in terms of what the NHS, as a massive and complex organization, could itself bear), subsequent years are almost certain to see not only an expansion in the number of Trusts but a clearer resolution of the freedoms and restrictions Trusts will enjoy. This is likely to err more on the side of freedom than restriction. The main incentives for Trusts are business incentives and the need to generate income. With relaxations in the restrictions of the first year of the reforms, new options will present themselves to Trusts.

Faced with a group of purchasers (DHAs and GP fundholders) with cash-limited budgets funded largely out of general taxation, and demonstrable unmet demand for health care, what should Trusts do? One clear option is to deal with increased demand by adjusting prices and/or to seek out non-NHS purchasers willing to buy surplus capacity. There have been a number of examples of Trusts using differential prices. In Manchester, the Christie Hospital offered purchasers the option of shorter waiting times in return for higher treatment prices. The offer was selective; only patients whose districts paid the higher price could take advantage of the shorter waiting times. The justification from the Trust's point of view was that without the additional revenue higher charges would bring, they would not be able to open a previously closed ward, in which case nobody would benefit. As it was, argued the Christie Hospital management, if some Districts agreed to pay the higher price the ward would be opened and some patients treated more quickly. Christie Hospital raised a notion from welfare economics concerning distributional optimality by stating that no one would be worse off and some would be better off if their initiative went ahead. The difficulty was that it ignored another economic concept – opportunity cost. Those Districts who paid the higher price would have less to spend on other services. That is, the benefit of shorter waiting times for a few is equivalent to the costs of perhaps no treatment or inferior quality treatment for others. In other words there is no such thing as a free lunch, or indeed operation. Although the Christie Hospital ran into difficulties with NHS purchasers over their idea, there is no reason to suppose that they would find the same problems with the private sector.

The Christie Hospital case suggests a potential for NHS hospitals to expand into the private medical market and hence tap into sources of finance other than that provided from general taxation and channelled via DHAs and GP fundholders. Laing (1990) suggests that one of the reasons Trusts will be able to take on the private health-care sector more vigorously than before is the change in consultants' contractual relationships with Trusts. One of the new freedoms Trusts have is the ability to directly employ consultant staff and to negotiate terms of service. Laing suggests that this could herald the beginning of a challenge to the traditional private fee structure for consultants, which could lead to substantial savings on private patient work for those hospitals who employ their own consultants (or who employ consultants to do private sessional work) – for example, Trusts.

Laing also raises the possibility of the development of 'preferred provider relationships'. This has echoes of the US-managed health-care movement in which tied relationships have developed between hospitals and third-party payers (sometimes they are one and the same). There is no reason to suppose that Trusts will not seek to negotiate preferred provider status with private medical insurers. Not only is this a way of entering the private medical market, but it also ensures some degree of long-term security for the Trust.

For hospitals like the Christie Hospital who, given a marginal injection of funds, can bring back into use previously closed facilities, possibilities exist for partnerships with the private sector. Such partnerships are not new to the NHS, but with the change in management and economic climate brought about by the NHS reforms they are likely to become more common.

The foregoing highlights a potentially very real trend over the coming years, namely, a growing breakdown of the demarcation between public and private health-care sectors. Whilst the 1981 review of alternative health-care financing sources looked at abrupt changes (to social insurance, or private insurance, etc.), the reality of the actual reforms of *Working for Patients* are likely to be for a more gradual erosion of current patterns of financing, with private-sector funds providing a greater proportion of overall financing than hitherto. The extent to which private financing 'crowds out' public financing (that is, the extent to which the increase in private-sector funding is offset by reductions in public-sector funding) is difficult to predict, however, and depends on decisions by the Government on levels of public funding, the demand for private medical insurance, the scope for private/public-sector collaboration, the extent to which regulation and control of the NHS is reinforced or relaxed, etc. This issue is dealt with in greater detail later on in this chapter.

Private provision and private financing

Whilst Trusts – still nominally within the orbit of the NHS – may find an increasing incentive to attract business and hence financing from purchasers other than DHAs and GP fundholders, their success at either establishing a foothold in, or expanding their share of, the private-sector market is by no means guaranteed. Indeed, competition with private providers may lead to a conscious withdrawal from certain areas of health-care services on the part of Trusts in order that they might concentrate on those services they feel better able to provide more efficiently and effectively, and where they feel they have comparative advantage. The corollary of this is a potential expansion of the private sector into these service areas.

What does this imply for financing? Depending on the services that are dropped, public-sector purchasers (i.e. those funded from general taxation, etc.) may decide to buy these services from the private sector, redirecting public finance into this sector of the health-care market.

Alternatively, if the new suppliers charge higher prices for these services, the cash limited public sector purchasers may decide not to buy from the private sector on the grounds that other, previously more expensive forms of care are now comparatively cheaper. The populations on whose behalf these decisions are made may take a contrary view, however, and decide to buy private health care in order to maintain their access to services previously bought by the public-sector purchasers. In this case, health-care financing from private sources (direct payments and insurance) will increase.

Public-sector purchasers – reassessing needs?

Similar changes may stem from initiatives taken on the purchasing side of the new health-care market. A major consequence of *Working for Patients* is the potential change in the purchasing pattern of DHAs and GP fundholders. Health Authorities have a responsibility to assess the health-care needs of their resident populations and purchase health-care services accordingly. In the first year of the reforms it was clear that needs assessment had been subordinate to the requirement to maintain existing patterns of service. However, as the stability restrictions relax, and as Health Authorities get to grips with the epidemiological mechanics of needs assessment and the consequent inevitability of trading off outcomes of alternative health-care services because of limited resources, purchasers may decide to reduce the amount of certain types of care they buy or, indeed, decide not to buy certain types of care at all.

Whilst purchasers may take the view (or be forced to take the view given limits on their available funds) that certain health-care services will not be purchased on behalf of their resident populations, the views of the resident populations themselves may be different. Depending on the strength of this difference and the ability to pay, there could be an increase in demand for private-sector medicine, if that sector is willing and able to satisfy this demand. With public-sector purchasers switching away from certain forms and patterns of care and perhaps investing in areas which have traditionally not been seen to be part of the remit of the NHS (for example, buying safety goggles for factory workers to prevent eye injuries rather than buying surgical services to repair injuries after they have happened), NHS providers may also seek to satisfy the demand for traditional forms of care by encouraging private patients.

Whether the pressure for change originates on the provider or purchaser side of the new health-care market, there is a distinct possibility that patients and potential patients may decide to take matters into their own hands and go private if they feel they are being denied access to certain treatments or forms of care they think they need. Whilst public-sector purchasers may be making rational and logical decisions as far as the community as a whole is concerned, these decisions do not always coincide with the perceived needs and desires of individuals, everywhere, all of the time. Although it has always (and inevitably) been the case that within a health-care system designed to serve the community as a whole, trade offs between the individual and collective good have been made, the introduction of new incentives into the system may sharpen and exacerbate (as far as individuals are concerned) these trade offs. There are counterbalances to this possible tendency, however. Purchasers are urged by *Working for Patients* to take more account of the wishes of patients and potential patients in their purchasing decisions. However, some of the traditional methods of accountability – Community Health Councils and representative Health Authority members – have suffered setbacks as a result of the reforms. Furthermore, whilst one of the reasons for creating trusts was to give local hospitals back to local people, in practice accountability is limited.

GP fundholders – potentials for cost-shifting?

Another set of key actors in the new health-care market are GP fundholders. The first wave of fundholders consisted of more than 300 practices, representing 1700 GPs, with over 4 million people on their lists and controlling over £300 m. of public money. In 1992–93, the number of fundholders is likely to double (NAHAT, 1991). For GPs willing to take on the rigours of managing not insubstantial budgets there are benefits in terms of the freedom to negotiate directly with hospitals and to influence directly the sort of care their patients receive. For virtually all GPs, talking to hospitals (in particular hospital management) about the services they want to buy, how those services are to be delivered, etc. is a new experience, as previous contact with the hospital sector was almost wholly routed through consultants. Budgets also give GPs the freedom of choice to spend their money as they see fit without the constraints of decisions about, for example, the local availability of certain services, which had previously been taken by hospitals and Health Authorities which many GPs felt ignored their needs. But now, GPs with budgets have the financial clout to make hospitals listen.

However, budgets radically alter the incentives faced by GPs. From a state of almost total ignorance about the costs of the care their patients incurred following referral and treatment in hospital, GP fundholders now know, if not the cost, at least the price of care for individual procedures. These prices may or may not reflect the true costs to hospitals of providing the one hundred or so procedures GPs are allowed to buy, but for the GP fundholder the prices hospitals charge represent a real call on their budgets. GP fundholders are now in the position of not only making clinical judgements about the care of their patients, but also economic or financial judgements about that care. This is a very new situation for GPs, and suggests that the way they make decisions about the care of their patients and, importantly, the outcome of those decisions, could be very different from previous practice.

One possible reaction on the part of GPs could be to encourage those on their lists (who could afford to do so) to purchase private medical insurance; in effect equivalent to shifting some costs of care – which would otherwise come out of GPs' budgets – onto individuals and private medical insurers. Why should GPs do this? Apart from the unlikely occurrence of private medical insurers signing up GPs as agents or giving GPs a percentage of premiums collected as a result of recommending people to an insurer, there are economic and possibly ethical incentives to shift costs. Faced with a limited budget (which may also underestimate the actual costs of referrals thought to be clinically necessary), fundholders may feel ethically justified in trying to reduce calls on their budgets so that they have more to spend on certain individuals or groups of individuals. Furthermore, GPs may shift costs in order to retain surpluses at the end of the year. (Such surpluses do not go direct into GPs' pockets, but can be used to invest in services, equipment, etc. at GPs' surgeries.)

The extent to which the take-up of private medical insurance increases over the coming years as a result of GPs' encouragement is impossible to predict. However, there would appear to be the incentive for GPs to promote private medical insurance, and with the prospect of growing numbers of fundholders, it would seem likely that there will be some, unquantifiable, increase in private financing of health care in the UK.

Tax relief on private medical insurance

It was widely believed at the time of the publication of *Working for Patients* that the decision to include specific tax relief on medical insurance held by people aged over 60 years was taken in the face of opposition from the then Secretary of State for Health as well as the Treasury. It is unknown what the Secretary of State's objection was, but the Treasury's was clear: such a policy would be costly. First, there were 'deadweight' costs, i.e. the costs of giving tax relief to all those now eligible who already had medical insurance. Secondly, there are costs arising from the increase in policyholders arising from the incentives the tax relief offers.

Although in theory virtually all people aged over 60 years are probably eligible for tax relief on medical insurance, and whilst there is a considerable potential market of uninsured over-60-year-olds (approximately 11.5 million in the UK), in practice there has been no significant increase in the take-up of insurance by this age group since April 1990 when the tax break was introduced. Part of the reason for this under-response probably arose from the fact that the policies the elderly would find particularly useful, such as coverage for long-term care, were comparatively underdeveloped in the UK. However, with increasing numbers of operators entering the medical insurance market over the last few years, it is likely that competition for business will produce more innovative and varied policies which are likely to attract this age group. Whilst this would counter the problem that some elderly, although perhaps attracted to private medical insurance because of the effective cut in price, either find themselves excluded from purchase on grounds of age or health status or cannot find any policy worth buying (because of restrictions on coverage, for example), it does not counter the problem that insurance may still be too expensive for most people.

It may well be the case that relief at the basic rate of tax is simply not enough of an inducement for most elderly to buy insurance. But given that the original intention of the tax break was to encourage the uninsured to obtain insurance, and not simply to help those who already had insurance and who presumably did not need any price-reducing incentive to buy insurance in the first place, what is the likely response to the apparent failure of the policy? There are three possibilities: scrap the relief; retain it; or extend it in some way. It was evident in the autumn of 1991 that there was some disagreement between the Department of Health (who seemed to favour the scrapping of the tax break) and the Treasury and other senior ministers (who favoured its retention).

Scrapping tax relief for medical insurance seems unlikely because of the objections it would raise from the insurance companies and provident societies as well as those people who currently benefit from relief. However, it could be retained in the hope that the private medical insurance sector responds by developing new and appealing policies for the over-60-year-olds such that new subscribers were attracted. But in this case it could be argued that it was not so much the tax relief that was the incentive to purchase insurance, rather it was the fact that the policies on offer were more attractive and perceived by subscribers to be of more benefit than previous policies. The third option would be to extend tax relief so that it had the intended effect of increasing the number of people with medical insurance. This could be achieved in a number of ways; for example, by increasing the size of the relief itself, or extending eligibility to all age groups, or dropping restrictions on employer-purchased policies, etc. Given that policy in this area has already crossed into effective subsidization of private medical insurance for one group in the community, there would seem to be no reason why the policy could not be extended, especially if this were to encourage significant numbers of people to buy medical insurance.

Overall, there would appear to be a number of ways in which private medical insurance could receive a boost as a result of the NHS reforms. But there are also a number of ways in which private medical insurance may be under pressure as a result of the reforms. For example, one important reason given by many people who buy insurance for doing so is their perception of shortcomings in the NHS, particularly waiting times. If the reforms make significant inroads into the waiting-list problem (even if this is only how the problem is perceived), then the benefits of insurance would be diminished and take-up consequently reduced. The balance would seem, however, to be on the side of increasing growth in private medical insurance, with the numbers insured by the end of the century, if not reaching half the population, certainly touching on 10 million – a 30–40 per cent increase on the current number of insured (*Health Service Journal*, 1990).

Alternative income sources

Whilst private medical insurance may be seen as the main alternative to tax financing of health care, there are nonetheless significant sources of funding for NHS care from patient charges, and to a lesser extent income generation and the sale of surplus assets. Although none of these sources of financing is ever likely to provide anything but a minority of funds to maintain and run the NHS, their contribution cannot be ignored. Overall, patient charges, receipts from asset sales and revenue from income-generation schemes in England were estimated to total nearly £2 bn. in 1990–91 (DoH, 1991). This is equivalent to 8.2 per cent of total NHS spending. The figure for the NHS as a whole in the UK is nearly £2.4 bn. Moreover, since 1981, these alternative sources of income have provided an increasing proportion of NHS spending. Despite the economic pressures on hospitals, the prospects for further growth in income from charges, asset sales and income-generation schemes are probably fairly limited over the next ten years.

Patient charges

Since their introduction in 1952, prescription charges have been increased 18 times – from a shilling (5 p) per form in 1952, to £3.60 per item in 1991. The real rise in the cost of prescriptions is around 300–400 per cent over this period. In the late 1960s certain groups were exempted from charges. The numbers who could claim exemptions had, by the 1980s, grown to about 31 million people, over half the population. Despite the increase in the number of people who are eligible for free prescriptions (around 85 per cent of all prescriptions currently cashed are exempt from charges) and a concomitant fall of nearly threefold in the number of chargeable prescriptions since 1970, revenue from charges has increased. Moreover, since the beginning of the 1980s, the number of chargeable items fell from an average of 5.3 per person to 2.9 in 1989. But even so, income from prescriptions continued to rise. Recent trends would seem to indicate, therefore, that charges could be raised further without reductions in income, even though the number of chargeable items may fall. Or will there come a point at which the additional income raised from further increases in charges is more than offset by reductions in the number of chargeable prescriptions cashed?

If prescription charges were merely to rise in line with inflation over the next nine years (assumed to be 5 per cent per year) then, by the end of the century each prescription item would cost nearly £6. But incomes would have risen also, probably enough to offset the effects of the prescription charge rise. However, if charges were to increase as they have done over the last ten years, then each item would cost nearly £20, equivalent to paying £13 today. Whilst even this level of charging may not prove prohibitive to the point of actually reducing total income, there is likely to be a significant fall in the number of chargeable prescriptions cashed, perhaps similar to the reduction of over 50 per cent that occurred over the past ten years. The political implications of the increase in charges and consequent fall in items dispensed is difficult to judge. However, it might be expected that there would be considerable opposition to such a rise in the price of prescriptions on the grounds that it would effectively deny access to treatment for those people unable to pay.

Similar arguments will apply to other areas of patient charges such as dental treatment and ophthalmic services. The latter service could provide an indication of future trends in prescription and dental charges, however. Rather than attempt to increase charges, one option may be to follow changes in the way ophthalmic services are paid for. Since 1985, there has been an increasing move towards the privatization of ophthalmic services. Currently, apart from some exemptions, all sight tests are now paid for directly by the public, and spectacles provided under the General Ophthalmic Services are only provided free to exempt groups (e.g. children under 16 years, glaucoma and diabetes suffers). As charges for prescriptions and dental treatment move closer to the actual cost of providing these services, so there could be an increasing tendency to argue that they might as well follow changes in the funding of ophthalmic services, i.e. effective transfer of financing out of general taxation and into direct payments by users of these services.

Income generation and asset sales

Income generation and the sale of surplus land, property and equipment, started to raise significant amounts of money in the early 1980s. Before 1980, receipts from asset sales were negligible, totalling a few million pounds a year, for example. Income generation schemes barely paid for themselves let alone generated any net income. Since 1982, asset sales have proved to be an increasingly important addition to the NHS capital programme. In 1988–89, asset sales in England totalled £271 m. – equivalent to nearly 30 per cent of the capital allocation for that year. Since then, however, slumps in the property market have reduced income from this source. In 1991–92, planned receipts were £240 m. – £60 m. less than expected. Recent estimates (*Health Service Journal*, 1991) suggested that the NHS would in fact only realise £200 m. Nevertheless, land and property prices will undoubtedly increase over the coming years, and the NHS will continue to divest itself of surplus assets. This process is likely to receive added impetus from the reforms. The creation of the internal market leaves providers increasingly cut adrift from a guaranteed source of income, and while health care remains the main line of business, providers will need to look more closely in future at all possible revenue raising activities, asset sales included.

A further incentive for reducing and rationalizing assets arises from the introduction of capital charges. Since 1 April 1991, owning capital assets (newly redefined as any asset valued at £1000 and over) incurs a cost which must be paid to the state. In the case of NHS Trusts, interest (and when possible, depreciation) has to be paid to the Department of Health on the value of the assets they inherited on becoming a Trust and also on any subsequent borrowings. For directly-managed units (DMUs), capital charges (interest and depreciation) must be paid to Regional Health Authorities. Although in the first year of capital charging the flow of money was purely nominal, representing no net addition either to the costs Trusts and DMUs incur, or effectively to the prices public-sector purchasers pay for services, in subsequent years capital charges will constitute a substantial proportion of both provider costs and purchaser payments. Trusts and DMUs with high capital charges are likely to find themselves at a competitive disadvantage compared with low cost units and will need to seek to reduce any unnecessary stock holdings.

Despite the vast size of the NHS estate (equivalent to nearly 30 000 football pitches), asset sales represent a finite source of income, and, judging from recent experience with fluctuations in property prices, one which no provider would want to rely upon too heavily.

In summary, whilst health care in the UK will continue to be mainly funded from general taxation, recent trends (for example, in patient charges) and the consequences of the NHS reforms suggest that other sources of funding, in particular private insurance, are likely to prove increasingly important.

LEVELS OF HEALTH-CARE FUNDING

If the sources of health-care funding are likely to change over the next ten years, what are the effects on total levels of funding? Does an increase in the number of private medical-insurance policy-holders mean, for example, that total health-care funding will increase? Two possibilities suggest that this is not necessarily so. First, increases in one source of funding may simply be cancelled out by decreases in another. Secondly, any idea that an increase in funding automatically means an increase in the amount and or quality of health care ignores the potential differences in costs associated with different forms of funding. Higher spending may merely be absorbed in higher prices. In looking at the prospects for levels of funding, therefore, trade offs between one source of financing and another, and differences in the costs of alternative ways of financing health care must be taken into account. Moreover, as one of the primary determinants of health-care spending is political (albeit informed by other determining factors such as demographic change, etc.), estimating future levels of funding entails some probably uncertain assumptions about future Governmental policy.

The size of the cake

Total spending on organized health care in the UK in 1989–90 was in excess of £32 bn. This included spending on the NHS, local authority residential accommodation, private and voluntary acute, nursing and residential care, pharmaceuticals, dentistry, ophthalmic services, etc. (but ignores spending on other, largely unorganized, health-related activities). Government expenditure plans for 1991–92 and recent trends in the increase in private-sector spending, suggested that total spending is now in excess of £40 bn. Whilst both public and private health-care sectors have seen real growth in spending over the last ten years, the private sector has grown more rapidly. For example, private spending on acute care rose by over 200 per cent between 1980 and 1989 (Laing, 1990), whereas spending in the hospital and community-care sector of the NHS rose by about 7 per cent (NAHAT, 1990b). As a proportion of GDP, spending on the NHS fell slightly between 1980 and 1990.

With trends indicating real rises in expenditure in both the public and private health-care sectors, what is the likely pattern for spending levels over the next ten years, in particular given changes in the health-care economy as a result of the NHS reforms and the consequent potential changes in funding sources?

As was noted earlier, past trends in public-sector funding of health care show generally increasing spending both in cash and real terms. A crude extrapolation of these trends would suggest a continuation of real rises in spending from now to the end of the century. However, there are a number of factors which need to be considered before drawing this conclusion.

As Bosanquet and Gray (1989) have pointed out, one important factor in Government decisions on spending levels – viz. changes in population size and age structure – suggests that spending should perhaps not need to increase as much as in recent years because of much slower growth in the number of elderly over the next ten years. For the NHS, the elderly (defined as people aged over 65 years) constitute its largest group of users. In fact, just over half of all NHS spending is directed towards this group (who make up just over 15 per cent of the population). Office of Population Censuses and Surveys' (OPCS) projections show little or no increase in the proportion of elderly in the population between 1991 and 2001. However, the relationship between population changes and health-care expenditure is more complex than a simple one-to-one correlation. When changes in the whole population structure are looked at, and when changes in the use made of the NHS by different age groups is taken into account, as well as consideration of predicted increases in the efficiency with which the NHS treats patients, projected spending based on demographic changes starts to appear more complicated. Bosanquet and Gray estimate that taking into account all these factors, NHS expenditure would need to rise by about 1 per cent in real terms each year between 1988 and 1995. Growth between 1995 and the end of the century would need to rise by a slightly lower annual rate, however.

Despite indications of rising demand and consequent pressures to spend more on health care in real terms, there is no automatic process which means that either more money will be spent, or that, if it is, it will necessarily be spent by the state out of general taxation.

Given the increased possibilities for alternative sources of financing for health care following the NHS reforms, there may be an increasing tendency at national level to trade off tax-funding against other sources of funding, especially with other competing pressures on public spending. This would reduce, perhaps to zero, any net increase in total health-care funding. One example of this practice is the way cost-improvement programme (CIP) savings were treated by the Treasury in its bilateral negotiations with the Department of Health over NHS budgets. Whilst it is difficult to prove that anticipated savings from CIPs were overtly traded-off against allocations given the closed process of bidding and negotiation that takes place at national level between spending departments and the Treasury, it is widely believed to be the case by those responsible for ensuring that CIP savings are made. Even if there is no overt trade off between planned savings and allocations, in practice planned CIPs are not ringfenced or protected in any way, and so knowledge of CIP targets must influence negotiations for NHS budgets in some way. A more overt, if implicit, trade off between CIPs and allocations has occurred in the past due to instructions to District Health Authorities from the Department of Health for authorities to use part of their savings to meet the deliberately underfunded gap between central government allocations for doctors' and nurses' Review Body pay awards and the actual cost of the awards. A recent example of a trade off between receipts from asset sales and allocations is implied by the fact that lower than anticipated receipts in 1991–92 led to a compensatory increase in capital allocations.

Trade offs may occur in other ways. For example, the privatization of ophthalmic services means that the NHS no longer needs to spend money on spectacles and sight tests (except for some exempt groups). Similar possibilities may arise with other services such as dentistry as noted earlier. As well as possible withdrawals from certain service areas, as private medical insurance becomes more popular there may be an increasing pressure on the Government to allow limited forms of opting out of NHS services on the grounds that it is unfair for those with insurance to continue to pay for services they do not use. (This would parallel one argument used to support the introduction of the community charge or poll tax, namely, that under the previous rating system, the majority of services provided by local authorities were consumed by people who had not contributed to their costs.)

Also, given the optimistic view of the private medical-insurance sector, with predictions for growth over the next ten years ranging from 30 to over 200 per cent (*Health Service Journal*, 1990) – equivalent to between one-fifth and one-half of the population holding medical insurance by the end of the century – it is hard to see the Government (perhaps any government) maintaining the current proportion of its tax revenue devoted to health care.

Finally, it is worth noting some possibilities regarding the funding of public-sector purchasers within the newly introduced internal market. In the first year of the reforms, purchasers were largely funded on the basis of previous years' referral patterns and previous years' levels of provider costs. That is, purchasers were given enough money to buy levels of service which more or less equate with past provision to their resident populations. The expectation is that the internal market will, through a process of controlled and regulated competition, drive down providers' costs. If this turns out to be the case, then one option for government could be to reduce funding to purchasers in line with reductions in costs of service. In essence, this is the same as the trade offs which are thought to occur with CIPs in the past. A successful internal market may thus not turn out to be an effective argument for increased funding for the NHS, but quite the opposite, implying a reproportioning of various sources of health-care financing away from general taxation.

9

CONCLUSIONS

The current reforms of the NHS in the UK cannot be viewed as anything other than massive and significant. On this point most commentators are agreed. A problem arises with speculation as to the eventual outcome of the reforms, however. The avowed aims of the reforms are uncontroversial: in essence, to make the NHS more efficient – a goal with which it is difficult to disagree. However, there has been (and remains) considerable disagreement over the reasons and necessity for the reforms, their diagnosis of the ills of the NHS and hence their prescription, and also their real intention. Much of the change the NHS has undergone and is continuing to experience, has been managerial. That is, it has been concerned with structures, hierarchy and managerial accountability. But at the reforms' heart lie some fundamental changes in the way the NHS is financed and the way in which it deals with its resources.

Some of the reforms in financing are obvious and immediate: the first moves towards capitation funding for Health Authorities as a result of the introduction of the internal market (or managed competition), for example. Others are less obvious and more long term: the increase in the proportion of private financing of health care as a result of tax relief and changes in the economic imperatives for NHS providers, for example. It is clear, however, that issues as fundamental as the right level of funding for health care and the equitable distribution of resources within health care have not been solved at a stroke with the implementation of the NHS and Community Care Act in 1990. Of the thousands of legislative and policy changes undertaken by governments, very few, if any, survive in their original form, or produce the exact change anticipated at their inception. The NHS reforms are amongst the greatest and most complicated of any. Not only do they deal with a very large and – managerially, financially and politically – complex organization, but they entail significant changes in the incentives faced by groups and individuals within (and outside) the NHS. This makes any prediction of the outcome of the reforms extremely difficult, and was one of the main reasons for calls for trials of the reforms before their full implementation. This book has attempted to highlight some of the possible consequences of both the obvious and less obvious reforms, with a view to making some predictions about the eventual, if not destination, at least course, health care in the UK will take as a result of the change it is currently undergoing. This final chapter draws together some of the themes noted in earlier chapters. In particular, it highlights some of the central financial issues/proposals raised by the reforms of the NHS, the probability of an increasing emergence of financial pluralism in health care and some of the consequences of the reforms for equity in health-care financing.

THE REFORMS AND HEALTH-CARE FINANCING

The NHS reforms are not the only changes the NHS has undergone in the last 10–15 years. However, in many ways this latest set of reforms are qualitatively and quantitatively more extensive and certainly more far reaching than any that have gone before. Whereas previous reforms such as the abolition of Area Health Authorities (AHAs), and the introduction of general management were by and large restructuring of particular parts of the NHS organization, the present reforms reach into all areas of the work, organization and finance of the NHS. (Ironically, the new incentives on the purchasing side of the pseudo market are now leading to the creation of purchasing consortia which often mimic the boundaries of the old AHAs.) The changes also introduce new incentives designed specifically to alter the way the service is run. Many of the most significant reforms are finance-based, affecting the health-care economy, and these are outlined below.

A quasi market in health care

A key change has been the separation of the provision of health care from the purchase of health care – a necessary (although, it should be noted, not wholly sufficient) step in creating a market in health care. The hope is that through a form of managed competition between providers, purchasers (and by implication, patients) will benefit from reduced costs of care, increased choice and higher quality of care – in short, all the benefits traditionally asserted to arise from market competition. Although this new health-care market is highly regulated (not unlike many other markets, of course), the enforced separation of providers from a guaranteed source of income will, it has been claimed, encourage providers to be more efficient, keep down costs and enhance quality in order to attract and retain contracts with purchasers. This represents a significant elevation of the principles of economy and efficiency within the guiding ethos of the NHS. Whilst the importance of such principles cannot be denied, their increased status raises the question of potential trade offs and clashes with other guiding principles such as equality of access. Already the notion of a 'fast-track' service has become a reality as a result of some providers offering quicker treatment to patients of GP fundholders in order to gain their custom, for example.

The introduction of managed competition has raised many questions, the answers to which will remain speculative until more experience has been gained in the way the new financial incentives affect the behaviour of the key actors in the new system. For example, it is still not clear how far the financial imperative (i.e. the need to attract contracts in order to stay in business) will be allowed to rule the survival of providers. How 'managed' is managed competition? Whilst in theory market competition appears to produce the 'right' results in the long run, all the problems arise in the short run as markets struggle to reach the long-run position. And the 'short run' can be very long indeed, and transitional costs from short to long run very high, as is evident in all markets which need to adapt to changing circumstances. Will providers who fail to attract enough business be allowed to go out of business? And if not, what is the point of the new financial incentives? But if they are allowed to go out of business, how can we be sure that this 'market' decision is the right one? Will a balance between the roles of purchasers on the one hand and providers on the other, be attained to the benefit of both? Or are there to be losers in the system? Furthermore, the first year of the reforms was transiti[illegible] thrust of the reforms with regard to NHS Trusts and [illegible] ders, for example, is for all units to become Trusts and f[illegible] become fundholders, are some of the early signs of behaviour in the new health-care market ('fast track' for fundholder patients, for example) unrepresentative of future prospects?

Semi-autonomous NHS providers

The creation of a class of NHS providers – Trusts – with significant autonomous powers to determine their own financing and provision strategy, employment of staff (particularly consultants) reinforces some of the possible developments arising from the introduction of managed competition and the separation of purchasers and providers. The financial imperatives of managed competition are sharpened in relation to Trusts. In terms of the source of health-care financing, NHS Trusts will find themselves under increased pressure to seek out all forms of income, and not rely solely on traditional tax financing arising from contracts with public-sector purchasers.

Although still subject to overall public-sector expenditure constraints as far as the financing of capital is concerned, Trusts have the power to borrow from the commercial sector, a totally new source of financing for the NHS.

As with the new pseudo market, there are still questions concerning the limits of Trusts' freedoms and the extent to which they will be allowed to develop in their own way, regardless perhaps of any national health-care strategies or of any underlying principles of equity in health care. Moreover, whilst Trusts have been promoted on the basis that local communities should have more say in 'their' hospitals, one price of this decentralization may be a greater fragmentation of services and a loss of coordination, both in economic and health-care terms. Much depends, of course, on the balance between the halves of the market. Will purchasers have the financial leverage to impose their will on Trusts? Or will Trusts be in a dominant, essentially monopolistic position, able to dictate terms? And can it be assumed in such cases that it will be patients who benefit, and if so, whose patients – GP fundholders', private insurance organizations', DHAs'?

Subsidizing the private sector

Tax relief on medical insurance purchased by the over-60 age group has been introduced. As was noted in earlier chapters, although this policy does not appear to have encouraged significant numbers of new subscribers, there are reasons to believe that, over time, this tax break could lead to an increase in the number of people holding private medical insurance. However, as was also noted earlier, this will depend on developments in the private medical-insurance market and further government encouragement in this area through, perhaps, an extension of the tax break to other groups and/or the relaxation of qualifying criteria for the current relief. Nevertheless, tax relief represents a significant policy breakthrough which, it may be surmised, could facilitate further policy developments in this area.

30 000 level playing fields

Associated with the creation of a quasi market in health care and the establishment of broadly level playing fields between the public and private sectors, NHS providers now pay a price for acquiring and owning capital. Since the creation of the NHS, capital has been treated as a 'free gift' from the state. The introduction of capital charges aims to redress the perceived cost advantage NHS providers would have over private-sector providers. A further aim of this reform is to increase cost consciousness amongst NHS decision-makers concerning capital investments. The ramifications of the introduction of capital charges are difficult to assess as the full mechanics of the process remain unclear for future years. However, by increasing NHS providers' costs (and hence prices for their services), capital charges may make private-sector health care a more attractive buy for public-sector purchasers.

Capital charges are likely to speed up recent trends in disposal of surplus assets as units with high capital charges attempt to cut their costs to become more competitive. For some units, however, rationalization of their capital stock may need to be very radical indeed, possibly involving relocation to another site, if they are to retain business. The scope for asset sales is still estimated to be large (Audit Commission, 1991), with the NHS owning land equivalent in area to 30 000 football pitches.

PUBLIC/PRIVATE MIX IN HEALTH-CARE FINANCING

As earlier chapters have argued, whilst the reforms of the NHS did not include many of the radical changes some had anticipated or urged, such as the privatization of the Service, one important outcome of the reforms would appear to be the encouragement of the private sector in terms of both health-care financing and provision. Whether intentional or not (although earlier references to unpublished reform ideas coupled with the general tenor of Government public-service policy over the last 10–12 years suggests intention rather accident), an increased role for the private sector is an important development for the NHS. The private sector and the NHS are now facing significant changes in their incentive structure which may lead to significant changes in the balance of provision and of financing in the UK's health-care economy.

New incentives for public providers and purchasers

Public-sector providers, particularly NHS Trusts, are likely to find themselves under increased pressure to seek out alternative forms of income. Whilst this will include raising revenue from asset sales, income generation and other non-health-care activities, perhaps the most important alternative source of income will be private medical insurance. Some of the reasons for this, identified in earlier chapters, include the likelihood of continued resource constraints for public-sector purchasers, continued expansion of private medical insurance following new entrants to this market, a continuation in past increasing trends for higher levels and higher quality of care and financial encouragement to medical-insurance subscribers through tax relief. Moreover, there are possibilities for a new form of cost-shifting with respect to GP fundholders with the emergence of an incentive to promote medical insurance amongst their patients in order to reduce pressures on their budgets.

New incentives for the private sector

For private-sector suppliers of health care the reforms are probably difficult to assess. Direct and very possibly vigorous competition from the NHS could prove damaging to private-sector suppliers, especially if NHS providers attract one of the private sector's main sources of funding – medical insurance. Earlier chapters raised the possibility of preferred provider status (similar to developments in the USA), with NHS providers – especially Trusts – perhaps looking to cement such a relationship with some of the big medical-insurance organizations. Such relationships may appeal to medical insurers keen to tighten their grip on the rising medical cost inflation they have experienced over the last decade. Whilst the NHS reforms may induce some rechannelling of insurance funding from the private to public sector, there are also prospects for increasing the level of finance from this source through tax relief for policyholders aged over 60 years (and the possible extension of this reform).

Financial pluralism: blurring the line

Shortly after the loss to the Labour Party in a by-election of one of its safest seats in Wales – a by-election in which the reforms of the NHS were seen by many to have been the single most important issue of the campaign – accusations were made by the Government that the Labour Party had lied when it had asserted that NHS Trusts had 'opted out' of the NHS. Aside from party political rhetoric, the issue of whether Trusts were in or out of the NHS in fact reflects a wider issue concerning a blurring of the distinction between public and private sectors as a result of the reforms. Again, as in other areas of public-service policy, financial pluralism – for example, joint public/private-sector financing of essentially public-sector projects and services – has been encouraged in the NHS in the recent past and has received a boost from the reforms. The creation of the internal market relaxes the notion of two health-care sectors (public and private) as, on the one hand, NHS units (Trusts and DMUs) have a clearer freedom to provide services to the private sector, and on the other hand, public-sector providers, freed from responsibility for provision, and with a clarified role with regard to ensuring access to health care for their resident populations (or, for fundholders, the patients on their lists), now have fewer restrictions when it comes to buying health care from the private sector.

The question of whether NHS Trusts are in or out of the NHS is not as straightforward as some have implied since there is no single indicator which settles the issue. Ultimately, of course, the question is meaningless, save for the strength of its political and emotional power. Whilst the Secretary of State retains powers of appointment to the boards of Trusts, the whole thrust of this and other aspects of the reforms was to decentralize control, specifically management control of the affairs of NHS units. A legal opinion would probably suggest that, although part of the NHS, in essence Trusts are being allowed to act as if they are not.

EQUITY IN FINANCING

That notions of equity are at the heart of many debates about health care cannot be denied. Whether they should be at the heart of any discussion is perhaps another matter. However, at the risk of putting forward a circular argument, the fact that equity *is* at the centre of many discussions, or is more often than not an underlying concern colouring views of topics in health care, suggests that equity ought not to be ignored or sidelined as an unrelated or separate issue.

Chapter 5 discussed two notions of equity in relation to the finance of health care – vertical and horizontal – and noted that a 'fair' system of payment for health care was one in which more weight was attached to vertical equity, where unequals (in terms of ability to pay) were treated unequally (in terms of their contribution to the funding of health care). Work by Wagstaff *et al.* (1989) has attempted to compare the degree of equity in financing across a number of health-care systems in terms of the level of contribution for various income groups compared with these groups' pre-tax income. Overall, the UK system, dominated by payments from general taxation, appeared mildly progressive (i.e. the rich paying proportionately more than the less rich in terms of pre-tax income). In contrast, the US and Dutch systems appeared generally regressive. These results are not totally unexpected, reflecting the intuitive feeling that the insurance-based systems of health-care payment in The Netherlands and the USA are less 'fair' than a system, such as operates in the UK, which is funded from a comparatively progressive tax system and which is unrelated to health status.

Whilst it might generally be accepted that the financing of health care should treat unequals unequally, equity of provision is generally accepted to be fairest when there is equal treatment for equal need. (It is taken to be axiomatic that unequals will be treated unequally in terms of treatment.) It is clear, however, that equity in financing cannot be divorced from equity in provision. It cannot be presumed that a 'fair' financing method necessarily leads to fair provision.

Equity pre-reforms

In fact, as LeGrand (1982) and others (e.g. Hurst, 1985) have shown, in terms of socio-economic groups (SEGs), the NHS appears to have failed to provide equal treatment for equal need, with higher SEGs apparently receiving more health-care expenditure than their level of illness suggests they should. Wagstaff *et al.* have more recently suggested that this is indeed the case in the UK, and furthermore, that in The Netherlands there is less inequity of provision (despite the fact, as was noted above, that the Dutch financing system was less fair than the UK system). So, although the NHS has been financed in a mildly progressive way, in practice there has been a degree of inequity in favour of the rich in terms of the share of health-care expenditure.

Equity post-reforms

Looked at overall, inequity has always existed in the UK's health-care system, with not just two tiers of care, but many, depending on ability and willingness to pay for private treatment. Within the NHS, however, the ethos has been equality, irrespective of income or social status. That the middle classes not only generally enjoy better health but seemingly disproportionate use of the NHS is perhaps less related to the system *per se*, as to social forces operating *vis-à-vis* the social class of doctors and the way they relate to patients, the level of medical knowledge of patients, etc. This is not to support the continuation of inequities that exist in the NHS, but to suggest that the system itself is not specifically designed to support and promote inequity.

The NHS reforms contain little if anything to positively tackle the issue of inequity in the NHS, either in terms of making the financing of health care even more progressive or in terms of reducing unequal treatment for equal need. In fact, the introduction of the internal market has already produced an example of an increase in *unequal* treatment. A number of GP fundholders have used their financial clout to negotiate quicker treatment for their patients. For GPs, doing the best they can for the patient in front of them, this makes sense. But at a wider level it raises questions of the fairness with which the whole community is treated. It is not only fundholders who (in the short term at least) appear to be able to improve access for their patients as a direct result of their ability to pay. District Health Authorities also have the prospect of cutting waiting times for selected patients, not on the grounds of the clinical condition of those patients, but through higher prices for treatment. Whilst such inequalities as a result of the reforms have been admitted by Ministers, the counter-argument is that in the long run the 'market' will distribute the benefits of shorter waiting times (to take one dimension of care) to all. However, it is not at all clear how this will come about as there is no inherent process within the new health-care market to guarantee such a redistribution.

BEYOND THE REFORMS

Prospects for the future financing of health care in the UK as a result of the NHS reforms are not easy to assess, as has been noted on more than one occasion in earlier chapters. However, there appear to be indications and tendencies which suggest movement towards financial plurality, with a continuation (probably accelerated by the reforms) of past increasing trends in private finance of health care, for example. Other sources of non-tax funding such as asset sales and income generation are also likely to increase in importance, although their role in financing will always remain limited. One consequence of an increase in alternative sources of funding may be an associated off-setting freeze (or reduction) in public funding.

The reforms of the NHS are by no means the end of change for health care in the UK, and, from experience so far, will certainly not be the end of debate about how the ABC economy of health care is organized. One certainty amongst the many uncertainties of the reforms is that they must be assessed and evaluated if lessons are to be learned and undesirable outcomes avoided. Whilst there are also lessons to be learned from the way other countries organize and run their health services – as has been discussed in relation to the West German and US systems – and particularly their experience of changes in their own health-care economies, ideas, organizational structures and economic incentives do not always travel well.

For the UK, the reforms of the NHS represent an essentially untried and untested set of policies, undertaken at speed and lacking any formal evaluation. Whether or not they will enhance Aneurin Bevan's view of a 'satisfactory' health service as one in which 'the rich and the poor are treated alike, that poverty is not a disability, and wealth is not advantaged' (Bevan, 1952) remains to be seen.

Ultimately, what lies beyond the reforms of the NHS is in the hands of future governments. Politicians will take the decisions which will affect the nature and substance of the way in which the NHS is to be financed, and the economic environment in which it is to operate (for example, free market, regulated market, public ownership).

The current reforms operate largely to change the economic environment (the 'internal market'), leaving the type and source of global financing essentially unchanged. (This is not strictly true as the funding of health care as a whole is not completely divorced from some of the effects of, for example, the creation of NHS Trusts.) Any future decisions about changing the new economic environment must be based on a proper assessment of the outcome of the present reforms. Future decisions about the global issue of financing health care in the UK will equally require assessment of current modes of financing and, importantly, an impeccable justification based on the American adage (which does travel well) that 'if it ain't bust, don't fix it'.

Any changes in the basis of financing (which, in the case of the UK, means a move to private insurance or social insurance or some combination of the two) will need to be justified in terms of the performance of the current – essentially tax-based – financing of health care. But international experience suggests that, at a minimum, a significant minority of the UK's population could not afford to obtain enough private medical insurance in order to guarantee current levels of access they enjoy under the NHS. With the US health-care system now becoming very unpopular not only with the public but also private medical insurers and health-care providers, it is not at all clear that the UK NHS should make any significant move towards privatization and fragmentation of funding on the scale of the US model.

Social insurance may appear an attractive alternative – but it may be only to those wrestling with the inconsistencies, unreliability, inequity, overproduction, poor coverage and cost inflation apparently inherent in such health-care systems as exist in the USA. For the UK, the advantages of moving to a system of health-care financed from social insurance are much less clear cut – and this is before taking account of the (transitional) costs involved in making the move.

Health-care policymakers are probably best advised to accept that health care is a social issue which benefits from substantial government involvement – not just in terms of policy coordination, but also with regard to the control of financing through the comparatively efficient means of taxation. Whilst opponents may argue that this arrangement is likely to encourage inefficiency of production of health care and downgrade freedom of choice for users of the health-care system, it is worth noting that after some decades of wrestling with exactly these problems, the USA is now starting to seriously consider forms of unitary purchasing of health care which fall somewhere between the dominant European social insurance and the (pre-reform) UK NHS models. In essence, any system will necessarily involve trade offs between conflicting policy goals (greater efficiency vs. greater equity, for example). The growing feeling in the USA is that not only have the trade offs now become unacceptable in social terms (lack of cover for millions of the population) but that trade offs between efficiency and equity have also broken down with escalating costs *and* decreasing equity.

Finally, perhaps the most crucial point of note for policymakers – and one which has received a greater prominence as a result of the reforms of the NHS, most notably the separation of purchasing and providing – is a redefinition of the issue of financing health care, namely, a shift of focus towards the financing of health *per se*. With this altered perception comes the possibility of facing up to some of the fundamental problems and issues of financing, such as the appropriate level of financing of health care, the balance of financing between 'organized' health care (for example, hospitals) and health-enhancing activities and programmes (for example, lower speed limits on roads, greater use of protective gear in factories) and the balance of financing between efficient health-care programmes and inefficient but socially desirable programmes. It is with this broader view of the financing of health care that the UK NHS can take advantage of the reforms it is now undergoing to begin to tackle the central issues and dilemmas in health care.

REFERENCES

Abel-Smith, B. and Titmuss, R.M. (1956) *The Costs of the National Health Service in England and Wales*. Cambridge University Press, Cambridge.

Altensetter, C. (1986) 'Reimbursement policy of hospitals in the Federal Republic of Germany'. *International Journal of Health Planning and Management*, **1**, 189–211.

Audit Commission (1991) *NHS Estate Management and Property Maintenance*. HMSO, London.

Bevan, A. (1952) *In Place of Fear*. Heinemann, London.

Bosanquet, N. and Gray, A. (1989) *Will You Still Love Me?: New Opportunities for Health Services for Elderly People in the 1990s and Beyond*. Research Paper 2. National Association of Health Authorities, Birmingham.

Campbell, J. (1987) *Nye Bevan and the Mirage of British Socialism*. Weidenfeld and Nicolson, London.

Chassim, M. *et al.* (1987) 'Does inappropriate use explain geographical variations in the use of health care services?' *Journal of the American Medical Association*, **258**(18), 2533–2537.

Cozens-Hardy, J. (1980) 'Hospitals are for patients'. In: Seldon, A. (ed.) *The Litmus Papers*. Centre for Policy Studies, London.

Culyer, A.J. (1976) *Need and the National Health Service: Economics and Social Choice*. Martin Robertson, London.

Culyer, A.J. (1989) 'The normative economics of health care finance and provision'. *Oxford Review of Economic Policy*, **5**(1), 34–58.

Culyer, A.J. (1990) 'Cost containment in Europe'. In: *Health Care Systems in Transition: The Search for Efficiency*. Social Policy Studies No. 7. OECD, Paris.

Department of Health (1989) *Working for Patients*. HMSO, London.

Department of Health (1991) *The Government's Expenditure Plans 1991–92 to 1993–94: Departmental Report*. Cmnd 1513. HMSO. London.

Evans, R.G. (1974) 'Supplier-Induced Demand: some empirical evidence and implications'. In: Perlman, M. (ed.) *The Economics of Health and Medical Care*. Macmillan, London.

Fuchs, V. (1988) 'The "competition" revolution in health care'. *Health Affairs*, **7**(3), 5–24.

Gerdtham, U., Anderson, F., Sogaard, J. and Jonsson, B. (1988) *Economic Analysis of Health Care Expenditures: A Cross-Sectional Study of the OECD Countries*. CMT Rapport 1988:9. Centre for Medical Technology Assessment, Linköping, Sweden.

Green, D.G. (1988) *Everyone a Private Patient: An Analysis of the Structural Flaws in the NHS and how they could be Remedied*. Institute for Economic Affairs, London.

Guillebaud Report (1956) *Committee of Enquiry into the Cost of the National Health Service*. Cmnd 663. HMSO, London.

Harrison, A. and Gretton, J. (1986) *Health Care UK 1986*. Policy Journals, Berkshire.

Harrison, S., Hunter, D.J., Johnston, I. and Wistow, G. (1989) *Competing for Health: A Commentary on the NHS Review*. Nuffield Institute for Health Service Studies, Leeds.

Health Service Journal (1990) 'Making a claim for private insurance', 4 October 1990, 1466.

Health Service Journal (1991) 'Land sales less than expected', January.

Hencke, K-D. (1990) Response to Jonsson, B., 'What can Americans learn from Europeans? In: *Health Care Systems in Transition: The Search for Efficiency*. OECD, Paris.

Higgins, J. (1988) *The Business of Medicine: Private Health Care in Britain*. Macmillan, London.

Hilman, A.L. (1987) 'Financial incentives for physicians in HMOs'. *New England Journal of Medicine*, **317**(27), 1743–1848.

Honigsbaum, F. (1989) *Health, Happiness and Security: The Creation of the National Health Service*. Routledge, London.

Horne, D. (1984) 'A survey of patients in the private sector'. *Hospital and Health Services Review*, March, 1984.

House of Commons (1972) *Fourth Report from the Expenditure Committee, Session 1971–1972, National Health Service Facilities for Private Patients*. HMSO, London.

House of Commons (1990) *Public Expenditure on Health Matters: Memorandum of Evidence from the Department of Health Session 1989–90*. Cmnd 484. HMSO, London.

Hurst, J. (1985) *Financing Health Care in the US, Canada and Britain*. King's Fund Institute, London.

Iglehart, J.K. (1991) 'Health policy report: Germany's health care system'. *New England Journal of Medicine*, **324**, 503–508.

Illich, I. (1977) *Limits to Medicine*. Penguin, Harmondsworth.

King's Fund Institute (1988) *Health Finance: Assessing the Options*. Briefing Paper 4. King's Fund Institute, London.

Klein, R. (1991) 'On the Oregon trail: rationing health care'. *British Medical Journal*, **302**, 1–2.

Laing, W. (1989) *Laing's Review of Private Healthcare 1989/90*. Laing and Buisson, London.

Laing, W. (1990) *Laing's Review of Private Healthcare 1990/91*. Laing and Buisson, London.

LeGrand, J. (1982) *The Strategy of Equality*. Allen & Unwin, London.

Leu, R.R. (1986) 'The public–private mix and international health care costs'. In: Culyer, A.J. and Jonsson, B. (eds) *Public and Private Health Services: Complementarities and Conflicts*. Basil Blackwell, Oxford.

Long, S. and Welch, W. (1988) 'Are we containing costs or pushing on a balloon?' *Health Affairs*, **7**(4), 113–117.

Ludbrook, A. and Maynard, A. (1988) *The Funding of the National Health Service: What is the Problem and is Social Insurance the Answer?* Discussion Paper 39. Centre for Health Economics, University of York.

Luft, H.S. (1981) *HMOs: Dimensions of Performance*. Wiley, New York.

Manning, W.G., Leibowitz, A., Goldberg, G.A., Rogers, W.H. and Newhouse, J.P. (1984) 'A controlled trial of a pre-paid group practice on use of services'. *New England Journal of Medicine*, **310**(23), 1505–1510.

Maxwell, R.J. (1981) *Health and Wealth: An International Study of Health Care Spending*. Lexington, MA.

Maxwell, R.J. (1988) 'Financing health care; lessons from abroad'. *British Medical Journal*, **296**, 1423–1426.

Maynard, A. and Bosanquet, N. (1986) *Public Expenditure on the NHS: Recent Trends and Future Prospects*. Institute of Health Services Management, London.

Mayston, D. (1990) 'NHS resourcing: a financial and economic analysis'. In: Culyer, A.J., Maynard, A.K. and Posnett, J.W. *Competition in Health Care: Reforming the NHS*. Macmillan, London.

Merril, J. and McLaughlin, C. (1986) 'Competition vs. regulation: some empirical evidence'. *Journal of Health Politics, Policy and Law*, **10**(4), 613–623.

Moore, S. (1979) 'Cost containment through risk sharing by primary care physicians'. *New England Journal of Medicine*, **300**, 1359–1362.

NAHAT (1990a) *Autumn Survey of the Financial Position of District Health Authorities 1990*. National Association of Health Authorities and Trusts. Birmingham.

NAHAT (1990b) *Healthcare Economic Review 1990*. National Association of Health Authorities and Trusts, Birmingham.

NAHAT (1991) *Spring Survey of the Financial Position of District Health Authorities*. NAHAT, Birmingham.

Nuffield Institute of Health Services Management (1989) *Working Party on Alternative Delivery and Funding of Health Services*. IHSM, London.

OECD (1989) *Health Data File*. Directorate for Social Affairs, Manpower and Education. OECD, Paris.

Office of Health Economics (1990) *Compendium of Health Statistics: 1989*. OHE, London.

O'Higgins, M. (1987) *Health Spending: A Way of Sustainable Growth*. Institute of Health Services Management, London.

Orros, G. (1988) *The Potential Role of Private Health Insurance*. Working Paper 6, Working Party on Alternative Delivery and Funding of Health Services. Institute of Health Services Management, London.

Parkin, D. (1989) 'Comparing health service efficiency across countries'. *Oxford Review of Economic Policy*, **5**(1), 75–88.

Parkin, D., McGuire, A. and Yule, B. (1987) 'Aggregate health care expenditures and national income: is health care a luxury good?' *Journal of Health Economics*, **6**, 109–127.

Pauly, M. (1988) 'Efficiency, equity and costs in the U.S. health care system'. In: Havighurst, C.C. *et al.* (eds) *American Health Care: What are the Lessons for Britain?* Institute for Economic Affairs, London.

Propper, C. and Maynard, A.K. (1989) *The Market for Private Health Care and the Demand for Private Insurance in Britain*. Discussion Paper 53. Centre for Health Economics, University of York.

Propper, C. and Upward, R. (1990) *A Micro-Simulation Model for Health Care Expenditure Forecasts*. Personal communication.

Reinhardt, U. (1991) *Bringing Out the Worst in People: The Corrosive Effect of American Health Insurance*. National Academy of Social Insurance, Washington DC.

Robinson, J. and Luft, H. (1988) 'The impact of hospital market structure on patient volume, average length of stay and cost of care'. *Journal of Health Economics*, **4**(4), 333–356.

Robinson, R. (1990) *Competition and Health Care: A Comparative Analysis of UK Plans and U.S. Experience*. Research Report 6. King's Fund Institute, London.

Rosenberg, P. (1986) 'The origin and development of compulsory health insurance in Germany'. In: Light, D. W. and Schuller, S. (eds), *Political Values and Health Care: The German Experience*, 105–126. Cambridge, MA.

Sandier, S. (1990) 'Health Services utilization and physician income trends'. In: OECD, *Health Care Systems in Transition: The Search for Efficiency*. OECD, Paris.

Spitz, B. and Abramson, J. (1987) 'Capitation and case management: barriers to strategic reforms'. *The Milbank Quarterly*, **65**(3), 348–370.

Stewart, I. (1990) *Does God Play Dice?* Penguin, London.

Timmins, N. (1988) *Cash, Crisis and Cure*. Newspaper Publishing, London.

Wagstaff, A., van Doorslaer, E. and Paci, P. (1989) 'Equity in the finance and delivery of health care; some tentative cross-country comparisons'. *Oxford Review of Health Policy*, **5**(1), 89–112.

Ware, J.E., Brook, R.H., Rogers, W.H. *et al.* (1986) 'Comparison of health outcomes at a health maintenance organisation with those of fee-for-service'. *Lancet*, **i**, 1017–1022.

Weiner, J.P. and Ferris, D.M. (1990) *GP Budget Holding in the UK: Lessons from America.* Research Report 7. King's Fund Institute, London.

Wells, J. (1991) Personal communication.

Wilensky, G.R. and Rossiter, L.F. (1986) 'Patient self-selection in HMOs'. *Health Affairs*, Spring.

Zwanziger, J. and Melnick, G. (1988) 'The effects of hospital competition and the Medicare PPS Program on hospital cost behaviour in California'. *Journal of Health Economics*, **7**(4), 301–320.

INDEX